With the assistance of:

Julian S. Ansell, M.D.
Christopher R. Blagg, M.D.
Henry G. Bone, M.D.
Paul W. Davis, Ph.D.
Edward M. Eddy, Ph.D.
Robert A. Gutman, M.D.
Thomas L. Marchioro, M.D.
J. William McRoberts, M.D.
Leon A. Phillips, M.D.
Belding H. Scribner, M.D.
David P. Simpson, M.D.
Roy W. Skoglund, Jr., M.D.
Charles E. Stirling, Ph.D.
Gail E. Thout, M.D.

THE URINARY SYSTEM

An Integrated Approach

WARREN H. CHAPMAN, M.D.

Associate Professor, Department of Urology
The University of Washington School of Medicine

RUTH E. BULGER, Ph.D.

Associate Professor, Department of Pathology
University of Maryland School of Medicine

RALPH E. CUTLER, M.D.

Associate Professor, Department of Medicine
The University of Washington School of Medicine

GARY E. STRIKER, M.D.

Associate Professor, Department of Pathology,
Assistant Dean for Curriculum
The University of Washington School of Medicine

W. B. SAUNDERS COMPANY   PHILADELPHIA   LONDON   TORONTO

W. B. Saunders Company: West Washington Square
Philadelphia, Pa. 19105

12 Dyott Street
London, WC1A 1DB

833 Oxford Street
Toronto 18, Ontario

The Urinary System: An Integrated Approach   ISBN 0-7216-2490-1

Print No.:   9   8   7   6   5   4   3   2

PREFACE

This book was prepared to present an outline of anatomy, physiology, and pathology of the urinary system to medical students. It is intended to introduce the basic structure and function of this system and to correlate this knowledge with clinical diseases. In the field of renal and urologic disease, there is no paucity of large, comprehensive, and expensive textbooks, but there is a lack of smaller books which are useful to the medical student in presenting succinctly the necessary data for him to understand and evaluate abnormalities in the entire urinary system.

For the sake of clarity, we have perhaps oversimplified many controversial subjects and, in some instances, given only one explanation where several exist. There has been no attempt made to give a comprehensive classification of diseases of the urinary system, but discussions of those which are most common, or which illustrate clearly some physiological or pathological concept, although they may be rare, have been included.

The reader in search of further detail is referred to the following books which he or she will find helpful: *Diseases of the Kidney* (Ed. M. B. Strauss and L. G. Welt, Little Brown & Co., Boston, 1971); *Physiology of the Kidney and Body Fuilds* (R. F. Pitts, Yearbook Medical Publishers, Inc., 1968); *University of Washington Teaching Syllabus for the Course on Fluid and Electrolyte Balance* (Ed. B. H. Scribner, University of Washington Press, 1969); *Pathology of the Kidney* (R. H. Heptinstall, Churchill, London, 1966); *Urology* (Ed. M. F. Campbell, W. B. Saunders Company, 1970).

We are grateful to our many colleagues who have contributed so willingly and abundantly of their time, talents and knowledge.

Finally, we wish to express our appreciation to Mrs. Kimberly Knackstedt, Mrs. Wilma Leach, and Mrs. Maudine Wilson for their secretarial assistance. We are most appreciative of John J. Hanley, Associate Medical Editor of W. B. Saunders Company, for his constant encouragement and helpful suggestions. This recitation of a partial list of those we are indebted to impresses us with our inability to repay all we have gleaned from others, were we not able to say, as did Cervantes through Don Quixote, "If I have not been able to repay the good deeds I receive with other deeds, I put in their place the desire to do them, and if that be not sufficient, I make them public; for he that tells and proclaims the kindnesses he receives would repay them if he could."

WARREN H. CHAPMAN

RUTH E. BULGER

RALPH E. CUTLER

GARY E. STRIKER

CONTENTS

Chapter 6

A Clinical Approach to Diseases of the Urinary System...................... 229

Chapter 1

INTRODUCTION TO THE URINARY SYSTEM AND BODY FLUIDS

It is no exaggeration to say that the composition of the blood is determined not by what the mouth takes in but by what the kidneys keep.

Homer W. Smith (1895–1962)

It is not unreasonable to ask why we have a urinary system. The most fundamental answer to this question is to be found in the workings of the individual cells. The millions of chemical reactions going on within the cells in our bodies depend not only on temperature and on substrate and product concentrations, but also on both quantitative and qualitative intracellular ionic and water activities. There exists an optimum environment for these reactions, which is maintained despite slight variations in extracellular environment by active transport processes and selective permeabilities of the cell membrane. However, the transport processes cannot cope with wide changes in extracellular environment. Such changes alter intracellular composition sufficiently to impair metabolic activity and may, if drastic enough, cause irreversible damage or death.

Higher animals are able to function in a widely fluctuating environment because their cells are not directly exposed to these stresses. The immediate environment of these cells is called extracellular fluid (the so-called internal environment), which remains remarkably constant even though the external environment fluctuates widely. This constancy or *homeostasis* is effected by sophisticated regulatory and excretory processes of the cardiovascular, respiratory, and urinary systems which, in turn, are coordinated by complex neural and hormonal mechanisms. The role of the urinary system in this scheme is to maintain the proper extracellular fluid volume and the proper concentrations of the fixed (nonvolatile) solutes. By regulation, we mean the maintenance of some physiological parameter at a set level (say plasma Na^+ at 140 mEq/L), and by excretion we mean the removal of waste catabolic products and foreign substances from the body.

The kidney performs these functions and delivers the urine to a collecting and voiding system (ureters, bladder and urethra) which is responsible for protecting the kidneys against the adverse effects of infections or elevated hydrostatic pressure.

Paradoxically, the effort that has gone into understanding renal function has been greater than that directed toward an understanding of the collecting and voiding system, even though diseases of the collecting and voiding system are clinically more common than those that are primarily of the renal parenchyma.

BODY FLUIDS

Water Distribution.   The most prevalent constituent of the body is water; it constitutes from 45 to 80 per cent of body weight. This percentage depends in large part on the amount of fat present, since fat contains little water.

Body weight-body water relationships of infants and adults of various body types are given in Table 1–1. A 75 kg (165 lb) man of average build might, therefore, have a total body water equal to 60% of his body weight, or 45 liters. As shown in Figure 1–1, this 45 liters is divided within the body into two compartments, the intracellular compartment, which is about two-thirds of the total body water, or 30 liters, and the extracellular compartment, which takes up the remaining one-third, or 15 liters. The extracellular compartment is further subdivided into the intravascular or plasma compartment of about 4 to 5 liters and the interstitial compartment of about 10 to 11 liters. Actually, there is a third compartment, the so-called transcellular fluid, which consists of intestinal secretions and cerebrospinal, intraocular, pleural, peritoneal, and synovial fluids. The transcellular fluids represent less than 4% of total body water, and their composition in some areas (gut, brain, and eye) depends on active transport processes; therefore, they will not be discussed further.

The infant's body water is 70% (80% in premature infants) of the

Table 1–1.   Body water expressed as per cent of body weight.

BUILD	INFANT	ADULT MALE	ADULT FEMALE
Thin	80	65	55
Average	70	60	50
Obese	65	55	45

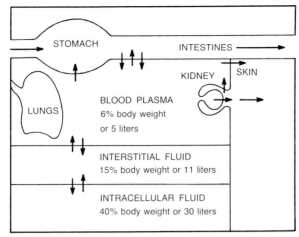

Figure 1–1. Fluid compartments of a 75 kg man of average build.

body weight. The relative size of the extracellular compartment in the infant is slightly larger (23% of body weight) than the 20% found in the adult. Plasma water is one-fourth of the extracellular compartment.

Measurement of Fluid Volumes. Although it is a useful approximation, the division of the body into gross compartments is certainly an oversimplification, since none of these compartments are homogeneous (cell water content, for example, varies greatly in different organs). The values quoted in Figure 1–1 are derived from tracer dilution studies. Some substances are largely excluded from one or another of these compartments; for example, labelled albumin is essentially confined to water or fluid of the vascular space. If one knows the absolute amount of albumin injected, one can calculate the plasma volume from the subsequent dilution of the albumin. Inulin and radiosulfate exhibit rapid capillary but slow cellular exchange and are used in a similar manner to measure extracellular volume (plasma + interstitial fluid). Intracellular volume size is estimated as the difference between total body water (as measured by tritiated water, for example) and extracellular volume. In clinical medicine, changes in body weight from day to day provide a useful indication of changes in total body water, from which changes in extracellular water can be estimated.

Transport of Water by Osmotic and Hydrostatic Pressures. When two solutions of different compositions are placed in communication with each other across a permeable membrane, there is a natural tendency for the two solutions to equilibrate. The driving force is diffusion, which is a manifestation of thermal motion. Equilibration takes place because in the region of higher concentration, molecules strike the membrane and pass through more often than in the region of lower concentration. This is true of solvent as well as solute molecules.

Thus, net movement due to diffusion occurs *down* a concentration gradient. Diffusion is the basic process for waste solute removal during peritoneal dialysis or hemodialysis.

More appropriately, one should use activities rather than concentrations, for activity is the tendency of one particle to move independently of all others present. When solutions are dilute, solute particles are far apart and concentration approximates activity. The addition of solute lowers the activity of the solvent by binding; thus, the addition of NaCl to pure water lowers the tendency of water molecules to escape from solution, and as a result both vapor pressure and freezing temperature are depressed. This holds for all particles in solution. Consequently, freezing point and vapor pressure depressions can be used to estimate the total number of dissolved particles in a solution. Measurement of freezing point depression is used clinically to determine the total osmotic concentration or *osmolality* of plasma, urine, and other body fluids. Actually, these measures give in effect the number of solute particles which participate in solute-solvent interactions. Those which participate in solute-*solute* interactions do not contribute to freezing point and vapor pressure lowering. Hence, these measurements are always lower than the true concentration of solute. The decrease in vapor pressure (ΔP) is given by the empirical relationship:

$$\Delta P/P = \frac{\text{moles of solute}}{\text{moles of solute} + \text{solvent}}$$

where P is the vapor pressure of pure solvent. The freezing point depression (ΔF^0) is given by the empirical relationship:

$$\Delta F^0 = K_f \times \text{solution osmolality}$$

where K_f(for water) $= 1.86°$ C/mole/kg H_2O.

If the freely permeable membrane previously described is replaced by a membrane permeable only to solvent (a semipermeable membrane), solvent will flow across the membrane until total solute concentrations or osmolalities are the same in both compartments. However, if a hydrostatic pressure of the appropriate magnitude is applied to the solution of higher solute content, no solvent flow is observed. The hydrostatic pressure raises solvent activity of the concentrated solution to that of the dilute solution. Evidently, the presence of solute can generate pressures; they are called *osmotic pressures*. The magnitude of the osmotic pressure (Π) between two solutions is given by the modified van't Hoff relationship:

$$\Pi = \alpha RT[\gamma_1 C_1 - \gamma_2 C_2]$$

where γ_1 and γ_2 are activity coefficients dependent on solute concentration and C_1 and C_2 are solute concentrations. The coefficient α varies with the kind of membrane, for it takes into account the fact that real membranes are never perfectly selective or semipermeable. Experimentally, osmotic pressure is the negative of the hydrostatic pressure necessary to prevent flow. Most biological membranes are highly permeable to water; therefore, initial osmotic differences between body fluid compartments rapidly disappear due to a redistribution of water. This fact is of importance in clinical medicine because measurement of the osmolality of plasma does accurately reflect the osmolality of all the body fluid compartments. Because the number of osmotically active particles inside cells tends to be constant, measurement of plasma osmolality provides a measure of intracellular volume or hydration and is used to determine the patient's need for water (see Chapter 4).

The phenomenon of *filtration* follows logically from the foregoing discussion. If a hydrostatic pressure is applied to the first of two identical solutions separated by a membrane, there will be a flow of solvent to the second. The flow of solutes will, of course, depend on the selectivity of the membrane. Those solutes which permeate the membrane only slowly relative to solvent will be concentrated in the solution under pressure. This increased concentration raises the osmotic pressure and opposes filtration. As discussed in the next chapter, the glomerular membrane of the nephron is a filtration membrane that is readily permeable to solutes up to a molecular weight of about 10,000 but increasingly less permeable to solutes of larger size. Thus, inulin (MW 5,000) is totally filtered while plasma albumin (MW 69,000) barely penetrates the glomerular membrane. Hence, as blood flows through the glomerulus, blood pressure produces an ultrafiltrate of plasma containing all of the small molecules, while the plasma proteins become more concentrated until a new equilibrium is established and filtration ceases near the venous end of the glomerulus. The rate of formation of this ultrafiltrate is a fundamental measure of renal function known as the *glomerular filtration rate* (GFR).

COMPOSITION OF BODY FLUIDS

Extracellular Fluid (ECF). The detailed composition of the body's fluids is depicted by the histograms of Figure 1-2. The dominant cation of the extracellular compartment (plasma plus interstitium) is Na^+, while Cl^- and HCO_3^- are the major anions. The excess of total inorganic cations over inorganic anions in plasma (20 to 22 mEq/L) is balanced by protein (17 mEq/L) and organic acid anions (5mEq/L). Plasma protein is largely albumin, which at pH 7.4 carries a net negative charge of 17, and since the albumin concentration is about 1 mM, protein contributes about 17 mEq/L to the plasma anions.

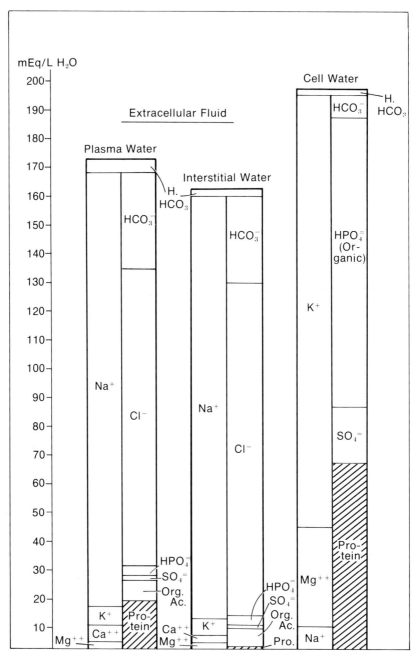

Figure 1–2. The electrolyte composition of body fluids.

Plasma Volume. The volume of the plasma compartment is of special importance because the integrity of the circulation is dependent upon maintenance of this volume. An important factor responsible for maintaining this volume is the osmotic pressure generated by the presence of plasma proteins in the vascular compartment and their virtual absence in the interstitial fluid. Most capillaries are permeable to small ions and molecules but are nearly impermeable to plasma proteins and larger particles. Hence, the interstitial space generally contains less than 1% protein. This low value of 1% is to be contrasted with that of plasma, which contains 6% protein. Since capillaries are highly permeable to water and small ions, one might suppose a uniform electrolyte distribution between plasma and interstitial fluid; however, such is not the case. The presence of protein in the plasma causes an asymmetric distribution of extracellular diffusible ions (mainly sodium, chloride, and bicarbonate) between plasma and the interstitium, as shown in Figure 1–2 and Table 1–2. This effect is commonly referred to as the Gibbs-Donnan equilibrium. This asymmetric distribution of ions is postulated to occur so that electrical neutrality will prevail. The negatively-charged albumin captures an equal amount of positively-charged sodium, thereby enriching the sodium content of plasma. Since the capillary is quite permeable to sodium, the sodium tends to diffuse down its concentration gradient into the interstitium; however, the electrostatic attraction of the impermeant albumin prevents the escape of sodium. Thus, a sodium diffusion potential of approximately 3 millivolts is established across the capillary wall. Chloride and bicarbonate ions, which are not similarly restrained, distribute in accordance with this potential. As may be shown experimentally and calculated theoretically, the net effect of plasma albumin is to raise the osmolality

Table 1–2. Electrolyte composition in plasma, plasma water, and interstitial fluid.

Ion	PLASMA mEq/L	PLASMA WATER mEq/L	INTERSTITIAL FLUID mEq/L
Cations:			
Na^+	142.0	152.7	145.1
K^+	4.0	4.3	4.1
Ca^{++}	5.0	5.4	3.5
Mg^{++}	2.0	2.2	1.3
Total Cations	153.0	164.6	154.0
Anions:			
Cl^-	102.0	109.9	115.7
HCO_3^-	26.0	27.9	29.3
$HPO_4^=/H_2PO_4^-$	2.0	2.1	2.3
Sulfate, org. acids	6.0	6.5	6.7
Protein	17.0	18.2	0.0
Total Anions	153.0	164.6	154.0

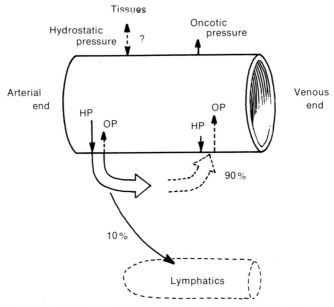

Figure 1–3.   Factors influencing fluid exchange in the microcirculation.

of the plasma about 1.5 mOsm/kg above that of the interstitium: 0.5 mOsm/kg from the increase in diffusible ions and about 1 mOsm/kg from the osmotic activity of the protein itself. This increase of 1.5 mOsm/kg is equivalent to a pressure of 28 mm Hg (1,000 mOsm/kg has an equivalent osmotic pressure of 22.4 times 760 mm Hg).

This extra osmotic pressure within the capillary causes an absorption of fluid unless it is opposed by hydrostatic pressure. However, if capillary hydrostatic pressure exceeds the protein osmotic pressure (also called colloid oncotic pressure), filtration of fluid into the interstitium occurs. Actually, both of these processes occur in the same capillary (Figure 1–3), as postulated by Starling nearly 75 years ago. At the arterial end of the capillary, where the hydrostatic pressure exceeds the protein osmotic pressure, there is a net movement of water from the vascular compartment to the interstitial space. Frictional resistance during the movement of blood through the capillary reduces the hydrostatic pressure, and at the same time, the concentration of plasma proteins is increased slightly because of loss of plasma fluid. At the venous end of the capillary, the plasma osmotic pressure probably exceeds the hydrostatic pressure and there is a net movement of water back into the vascular compartment. Under normal circumstances this entire process is finally balanced, with 90 per cent of the fluid which is filtered at the arterial end being returned to the venous side of the capillary bed. The remaining 10 per cent is returned to the plasma compartment through the lymphatics. It is clear from this schema that if the capillary hydrostatic pressure is excessive or the plasma osmotic pressure in the capillaries is deficient, then an excess of fluid can accumulate in the interstitial fluid; if the capacity of the lymphatics to remove this fluid is exceeded, then edema may occur.

Intracellular Fluid (ICF). Because cells in various organs differ, there is no typical intracellular fluid as shown in Figure 1–2. However, intracellular potassium is, with minor exceptions, the dominant cation; organic phosphates and protein are the major anions. The amount of chloride is variable but is always much lower than the ECF chloride. The osmotic activity of the polyvalent anions and the extent of ion and water binding is not known; thus, intracellular osmolality is uncertain. Nevertheless, the fact that increasing the concentration of extracellular substances such as sodium and glucose shrinks cells, while increasing the concentration of penetrating solutes such as urea expands cellular volume, suggests no large osmotic gradient between intracellular and extracellular fluids. To unequivocally answer this question, one needs to know intracellular pressure. The phenomena just described are the basis for the term *isotonic;* an isotonic solution causes no change in cell volume. Solutions of the same osmolality are *isosmotic.* Although all isotonic solutions are isosmotic to plasma, not all isosmotic solutions are isotonic. For example, an isosmotic solution of urea is not isotonic and will produce swelling of body cells. This is caused by penetration of cellular membranes by both solute (urea) and solvent (water). This example is clinically important because of the frequent occurrence of changes in the body fluid concentration of urea, which produce changes in osmolality but no differential shift of body water, as urea is rapidly distributed throughout intracellular and extracellular water.

Chapter 2

STRUCTURE AND FUNCTION OF THE HUMAN URINARY SYSTEM

Too much attention has been paid to the excretory offices of the kidney to the neglect of its conservative sources.

JOHN P. PETERS (1887–1955)

General. The urinary system consists of the kidneys, their ureters, the bladder with its valves, and the urethra. The kidneys control the composition of the body's fluids through a series of complex filtration and transport processes which modify solutes and water in the renal circulation. The final product, urine, is transferred by the ureters to the bladder where it is stored. Distention of the bladder due to filling initiates the micturition reflex, which voids the bladder of urine. The urine leaves the bladder via the urethra.

THE KIDNEY

Position and Relationships. The kidneys are situated in the posterior part of the abdomen in the retroperitoneal space, one on either side of the vertebral column, and are surrounded by a variable amount of fat and loose areolar tissue (Figure 2–1, FSA–1; Figure 2–2, FSA–2; Figure 2–3). The upper poles lie approximately 1 cm closer to the vertebral column than do the lower poles, with the long axes paralleling the psoas muscles. The upper margins are at a level of the upper border of the 12th thoracic vertebra and the lower margins are at a level with the 3rd lumbar vertebra. The kidneys are mobile during respiration and may move as much as 2 cm (Figure 2–4, FSA–3). In the adult male, the kidney weight varies from approximately 125 gm to 170 gm, while in the adult female, the kidney weighs 10 gm less. Although generally impalpable,

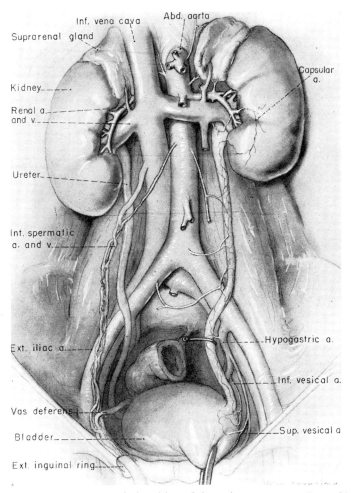

Inf. vena cava

Abd. aorta

Suprarenal gland

Capsular a.

Kidney

Renal a. and v.

Ureter

Int. spermatic a. and v.

Ext. iliac a.

Hypogastric a.

Inf. vesical a.

Vas deferens

Sup. vesical a

Bladder

Ext. inguinal ring

Figure 2–1 (FSA–1). Gross relationships of the urinary system. (From Urology, 1st ed. Vol. 1, edited by M. Campbell. W. B. Saunders Co., Philadelphia, 1954.)

the lower pole of the kidney may be felt in a thin individual in full inspiration during bimanual examination. Ordinarily, the right kidney is slightly lower than the left due to the presence of the liver; however, in approximately 15 percent of people, the left kidney may be lower. The kidney is roughly 11.5 cm (or 3 to 3½ vertebral bodies) in length, 5 to 7 cm in breadth, and 2.5 cm in thickness. Sex and overall body size must be taken into account in assessing renal size. The right kidney is normally slightly smaller and thicker than the left. Renal size is of particular significance in discussions of hypertension. Where a size difference of more than 1 cm exists, a renal etiology for the elevated blood pressure should be considered.

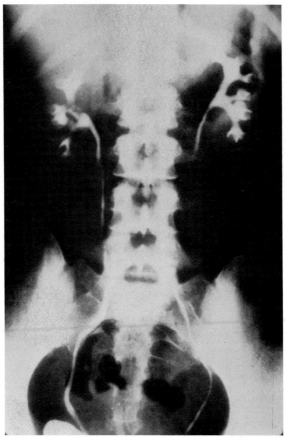

Figure 2-2 (FSA-2). Normal radiographic appearance of urinary system filled with contrast medium.

The kidney is shaped like a bean, with a concave medial margin containing a slit-like aperture called the renal hilum or hilus, through which pass branches of the renal artery and the renal vein, the pelvis of the ureter, lymphatics, and a small plexus of nerve fibers. The surface of the kidney is invested by a strong fibrous capsule, and external to this is surrounded by a mass of fatty tissue, the perirenal fat. This fatty tissue permits the kidneys to be seen on plain radiographs of the abdomen, since it is considerably more radiolucent than the kidney and the surrounding muscular structures. Surrounding the fat is a layer of renal (perirenal, Gerota's) fascia which forms an envelope around the kidney. This is a condensation of the retroperitoneal connective tissue and is a continuation of the fascia propria which reinforces the peritoneum. Around the kidney it forms anterior and posterior layers which unite above the kidneys and then separate to enclose the adrenal glands. Inferiorly it extends around the ureters. This fascia tends to limit or direct the spread of perirenal infections, hemorrhage, and the extravasation of urine.

The kidneys are in close relationship to other retroperitoneal structures. The medial portion of the right kidney is in contact with the liver. The liver and kidney, however, are separated by two layers of peritoneum. The lower lateral portion is related to the retroperitoneal surface of the ascending colon and hepatic flexure. The superior pole is covered by the adrenal (suprarenal) gland. The posterior surface is adjacent to the muscular diaphragm and the muscles of the posterior abdominal wall. The medial portion of the left kidney is associated with the tail of the pancreas and the lower pole with the descending colon. The superior pole is covered by the adrenal gland on the left side, and the rest of the anterior kidney surface is peritonealized by the colonic mesentery and is mainly related to the spleen. These relationships are of considerable importance from the standpoint of renal deformity and displacement caused by enlargement of the contiguous organs.

Gross Appearance of Renal Parenchyma.   If the kidney is bisected into dorsal and ventral halves and the cut surface viewed, the paren-

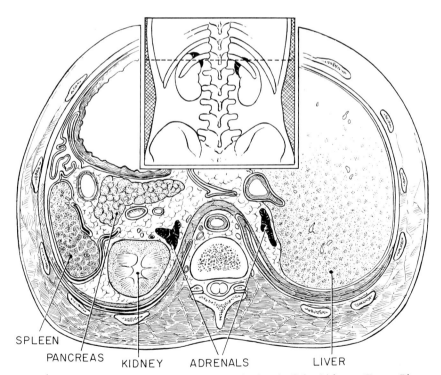

SPLEEN
PANCREAS   KIDNEY   ADRENALS   LIVER

Figure 2–3.   Cross-section of abdomen at the level of the kidney. (From Glenn, J. F., *in* Urologic Surgery, edited by J. F. Glenn and W. H. Boyce. Hoeber Medical Division, Harper & Row, Publishers, New York, 1969.)

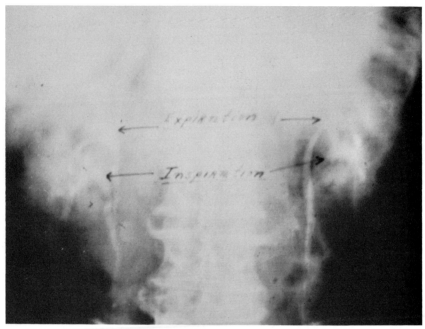

Figure 2–4 (FSA–3). Double exposure of excretory urogram, showing changes in position with inspiration and expiration.

chyma can be seen to consist of a dark red cortical portion and a pale medullary portion. The medullary portion is arranged into several cone-shaped or pyramidal projections separated from each other by sections of cortex called renal columns. The bases of the pyramids face the cortex of the kidney, while the apices point toward the renal hilus and project into the renal pelvis. The structural difference in the renal cortex and medulla results from the type and orientation of the units comprising these zones. The cortex of the kidney contains tubules and glomeruli, while the medulla contains only tubules. At intervals along the bases of the pyramids, perpendicular elements penetrate into the cortex. Although they are called medullary rays, they comprise part of the cortex. Each medullary ray forms the center of a small cylinder of tissue called a renal lobule.

The number of pyramids varies from 4 to 18, and the average number is about 8. The pyramid appears striated because it is made up of parallel tubules, some of which coalesce into larger collecting ducts. These larger collecting ducts pierce the apex of the pyramid. The apex is called the papilla. The large collecting ducts open into a receptacle called the minor calyx. The portion of the minor calyx which projects upward around the sides of the papilla is called the fornix and is important since the early signs of infection and obstruction occur here. Minor

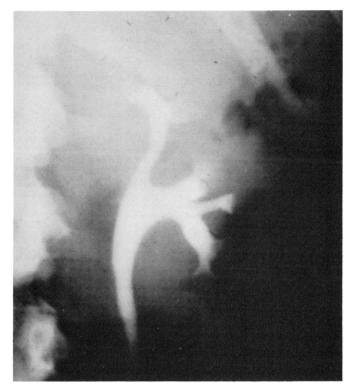

Figure 2–5 (FSA–4).   Excretory urogram with detail of calyces.

calyces unite to form major calyces, which may vary in number from two to four; usually three can be seen on an excretory urogram (Figure 2–5, FSA–4). The major calyces then unite to form a curving funnel, the renal pelvis, which bends caudally and medially to become the ureter at a point called the uretero-pelvic junction.

The calyces and the renal pelvis are lined by transitional epithelium. The surrounding smooth muscle is arranged in such a way as to propel urine to the ureters.

Renal Blood Supply.   The renal arteries arise from the sides of the aorta at the level of the first or second lumbar vertebral body (Figure 2–1). Accessory renal arteries have a reported occurrence of 20 to 30 per cent and usually supply the lower poles of the kidneys. The main renal artery as a rule divides into anterior (ventral) and posterior (dorsal) divisions in the hilum (Figure 2–6, FSA–5) which then divide into interlobar branches. The interlobar arteries course adjacent to the medullary pyramids and run within the renal columns. At the junction of the medulla and cortex, the interlobar vessels divide to form many arcuate vessels which course along the base of the medullary pyramid and

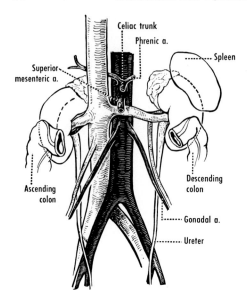

Figure 2–6 (FSA–5). Relations of kidneys and great vessels. (From Anatomy, Edited by E. Gardner, D. J. Gray, and R. O'Rahilly. W. B. Saunders Co., Philadelphia, 1969.)

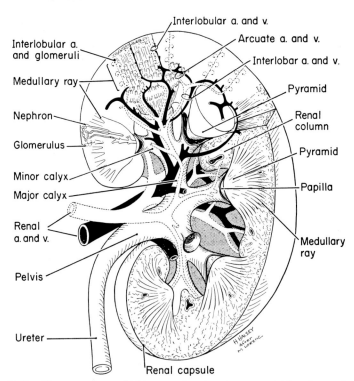

Figure 2–7. Cross-section of kidneys, showing intrarenal blood supply. (From Koch, A., *in* Physiology and Biophysics, 19th edition, edited by T. C. Ruch and H. D. Patton. W. B. Saunders Co., Philadelphia, 1965.)

give rise to the interlobular arteries. These latter vessels run perpendicularly toward the capsule half way between the medullary rays (Figure 2–7). Because they lie between the renal lobules, they are called interlobular arteries. The afferent arterioles arise from the interlobular arteries and supply one or more glomeruli. The afferent arterioles divide to form a branching capillary net inside each glomerulus and then merge to form the efferent arteriole. The efferent arteriole leaves the glomerulus and forms either the peritubular capillaries in the case of cortical nephrons, or the arteriolae rectae in the case of juxtamedullary nephrons (Figure 2–8). The arteriolae rectae are parallel, relatively unbranched vessels which extend into the renal medulla, where they give rise to capillary plexuses. The two capillary beds found in series

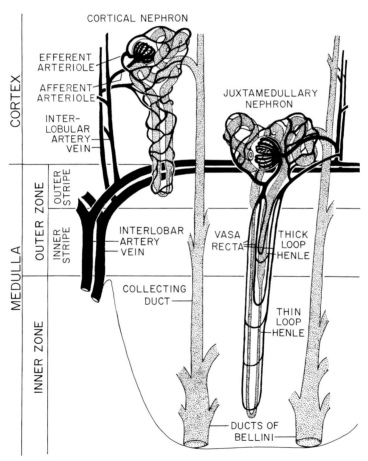

Figure 2–8. Diagram of blood supply to the nephron. (From *Physiology of the Kidney and Body Fluids* by Robert F. Pitts. Copyright © 1968 by Year Book Medical Publishers. Used by permission.)

in the renal arteriolar system comprise an arterial portal system similar to the venous portal system in the liver.

The veins are formed near the surface of the kidney by confluence of the capillaries of the cortex. The veins drain into the interlobular veins adjacent to the interlobular arteries, and become arcuate veins at the junction of the cortex and medulla. The venulae rectae in the medulla also feed into the arcuate veins, which then form interlobar veins. These empty into segmental veins, which continue from the anterior and posterior sides of the renal pelvis to form the renal veins. The left renal vein receives the left adrenal vein and the left testicular or ovarian vein before passing anterior to the aorta to enter the inferior vena cava. The right adrenal and right gonadal veins enter directly into the inferior vena cava. The left renal vein frequently receives the left second lumbar vein, which provides the intermediate root of the hemiazygos vein (about 25 percent of cases). The right renal vein is shorter and lies dorsal to the duodenum. Lymphatics have been reported in the capsule and around the larger vessels. They drain toward the arcuate vessels or to the surface capsule. The former converge near the hilus into six or eight channels.

Renal Blood Flow (RBF).   Because of its low vascular resistance, the kidney under resting conditions receives 1200 ml/min of blood, or

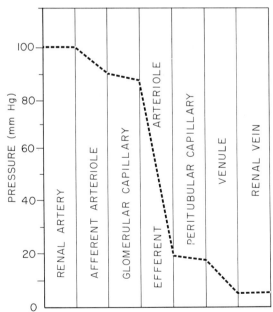

Figure 2–9. Pressure gradients in the renal circulation. (From *Physiology of the Kidney and Body Fluids* by Robert F. Pitts. Copyright © 1968 by Year Book Medical Publishers. Used by permission.)

approximately 25 per cent of the cardiac output. Intrarenal blood flow is not equally distributed; the cortex receives 93 per cent of the total RBF, although the cortex comprises only 75 percent of the total renal mass. Even within the cortex, blood flow is heterogeneous, with the flow rates to superficial and juxtamedullary glomeruli varying and dependent on neurogenic, hormonal, and metabolic factors. The 7 per cent of the RBF which perfuses the medulla is also non-uniform; the outer medulla receives the most, and only 1 per cent of the total RBF perfuses the papillary area.

The pressure gradients and sites of major resistance to flow within the kidney are illustrated in Figure 2–9. The major gradient across the glomerular capillary bed is produced by a relatively high resistance in the efferent arterioles. However, changes in renal arterial pressure produce proportional variations in the afferent arteriolar resistance, which tends to preserve a constant RBF and glomerular capillary pressure. This phenomenon of relative constancy of the RBF when mean arterial pressure is increased above 90 mm Hg is displayed in Figure 2–10. The correlative changes of renal vascular resistance with changes in arterial pressure have been observed in innervated, denervated, and isolated perfused kidneys, and is termed *intrinsic regulation* or *autoregulation*. Accordingly, it is generally accepted that autoregulation is the result of intrarenal mechanisms. Although the exact mechanism of this control is unknown, one of the most attractive current theories is one related to the operation of the juxtaglomerular apparatus; it will be discussed in a later section.

In addition to autoregulatory capacity, renal circulation is controlled by *extrinsic* (neurogenic and hormonal) factors. Renal vessels are richly supplied with sympathetic nerve fibers which are vasoconstrictive. In the supine resting state the output of the renal nerves is small, and tonic vasoconstrictor activity is negligible. In the erect position, vasoconstrictor activity becomes significant and increases with stress. However, the rate of filtration across the glomerular capillary bed varies little

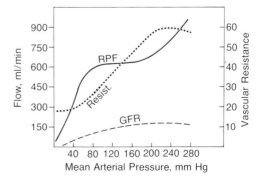

Figure 2–10. Relationship between mean renal arterial pressure and blood flow.

unless life is threatened by a severe loss of extracellular fluid; then both glomerular filtration rate (GFR) and total RBF are sacrificed in order to preserve heart and brain perfusion.

Humoral control is provided by circulating hormones such as epinephrine, norepinephrine, and angiotensin, which produce vaso-constriction. Attempts to differentiate renal vascular reactions into alpha and beta receptor-type responses have been unsuccessful. In contrast to endogenous hormones, certain drugs are effective in producing vasodi-latation. Serotonin (5-hydroxytryptamine) in low concentration pro-duces a significant increase in total RBF with a small reduction in GFR. Likewise, acetylcholine in low doses dilates renal vessels, as do papa-verine, aminophylline, hydralazine, and dopamine. Usually GFR does not increase parallel to the increase in RBF. This behavior may be explained by the dilation of efferent arterioles and the increase in intratubular hydrostatic pressure which occurs during renal vasodilata-tion. Although little is known about the action of the polypeptides such as bradykinin, they appear to have little effect upon normal control of renal hemodynamics.

Renal Nerve Supply. Each kidney has 10 to 15 small nerves (sym-pathetic) which enter the hilum, are distributed to the blood vessels, and produce vasoconstriction. These nerves arise from the renal plexus, which is formed by contribution from the celiac plexus, the celiac gangli-on, the aortic plexus, and from the lesser and lowest splanchnic nerves. The nerve supply to the kidney communicates with that of the spermatic plexus; this fact may explain testicular pain in afflictions of the kidney.

THE NEPHRON

Divisions of the Nephron. The basic functional unit of the kidney is the nephron, a long tubular structure made up of successive epithelial segments of diverse structure and transport function (Figure 2–11, FSA–6). A variety of names have been proposed for the nephron seg-ments. Consistent with current usage, the following can be distin-guished: (1) a renal corpuscle (Bowman's capsule and the glomerulus, a tuft of capillaries), (2) a proximal tubule (convoluted portion and straight portion), (3) a thin limb, (4) a distal tubule (straight portion, macula densa, and convoluted portion), and (5) a connecting portion of a collecting duct system.

The morphology of a specific nephron varies somewhat with its position in the kidney. Of the approximately one million nephrons in each human kidney, 7 out of 8 are cortical nephrons and have short loops of Henle with a short or non-existent thin limb segment. The remaining 1/8 are juxtamedullary nephrons with glomeruli lying near the cortical-medullary junction and having long loops of Henle with

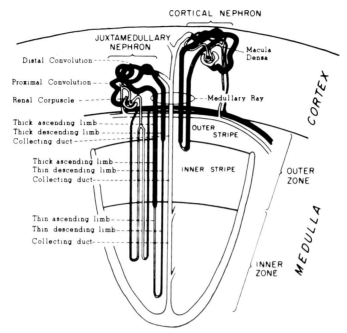

Figure 2-11 (FSA-6). Position of cortico- and juxtamedullary nephrons in kidney. (From Bulger, R., *in* Histology, 3rd edition, edited by R. O. Greep and L. Weiss. McGraw-Hill Book Co., New York, 1973.)

long thin limb segments. The zonation of the kidney, seen grossly, results from the fact that the same segments from all nephrons tend to lie in a given region.

The cortical substance can be divided into a convoluted portion and the medullary rays. The convoluted portion consists of glomeruli, convoluted portions of the proximal and distal tubules, and the connecting portions of the collecting ducts. The medullary ray is composed of the straight portions of the proximal and distal tubules and the collecting ducts. The medulla contains loops of Henle and collecting ducts.

Glomerulus

General. From its structure alone, one might surmise that the function of the glomerulus is one of filtration (Figure 2–12, FSA–7). The glomerulus represents an extensive capillary network, enclosed by a collection chamber (Bowman's capsule and space enclosed). This space opens into the tubular lumen of the nephron. The driving force for filtration is the hydrostatic pressure in the capillary. Regulation of capillary pressure, and hence filtration rate, is accomplished by intrinsic and extrinsic adjustment of afferent and efferent arteriolar resistances, while

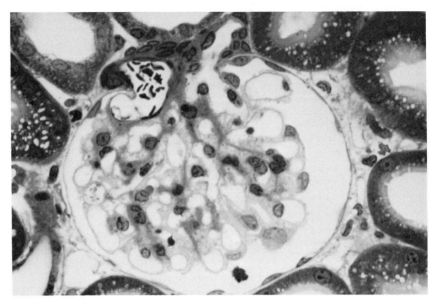

Figure 2-12 (FSA-7). Structure of glomerulus.

the composition of the filtrate is determined by the nature of the filtration barrier.

Bowman's Capsule. Bowman's capsule consists of a double-walled cup-like structure analogous to a balloon punched in with a fist. The

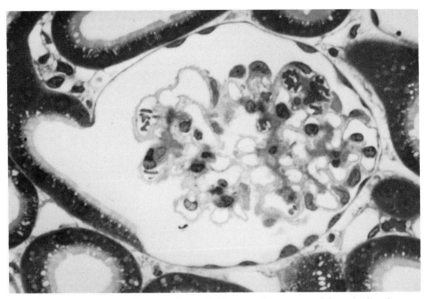

Figure 2-13 (FSA-8). Connection of Bowman's space with tubular lumen. (From Bulger, R., *in* Histology, 3rd edition, edited by R. O. Greep and L. Weiss. McGraw-Hill Book Co., New York, 1973.

space lying between the two layers is called Bowman's space (urinary space) and is continuous with the lumen of the proximal tubule of the nephron (Figure 2–13, FSA–8). The parietal or outer layer of the cup-like structure is formed by squamous epithelial cells and their basement membrane. The cells are shaped somewhat like fried eggs and are bound closely together by junctional complexes. The squamous cells and their basement membrane are continuous with the epithelium and basement membrane of the proximal tubule. A visceral layer forms the inner wall of the double cup-shaped structure and is made up of cells called podocytes. The podocyte is similar in shape to an octopus, with numerous large arms extending out from the cell body (Figure 2–14, FSA–9). These large arms in turn give rise to smaller processes (pedicels) that lie on the glomerular basement membrane and interdigitate with adjacent pedicels. The gaps or slits between adjacent pedicels are bridged by a thin layer of material called the filtration slit membrane. The glomerular basement membrane separates the visceral epithelial cell from the capillary endothelium (Figure 2–15, FSA–10).

The glomerular capillaries are lined by extremely attenuated en-

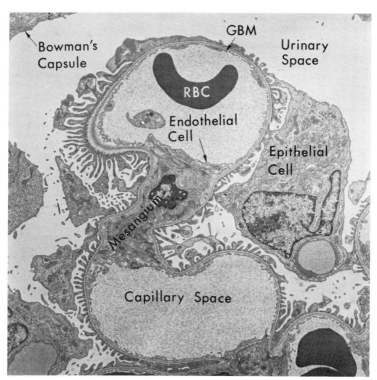

Figure 2–14 (FSA–9). Electron micrograph of glomerular capillary lumen, demonstrating position of podocyte (visceral epithelial cell).

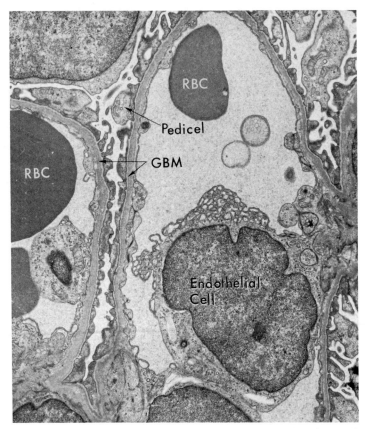

Figure 2–15 (FSA–10). High-power electron micrograph showing endothelial cell, glomerular basement membrane, and epithelial cell.

dothelial cells that are penetrated by frequent pores. The capillary endothelium lies on the opposite side of the basement membrane from the pedicels of the podocyte.

A third glomerular cell type is called the mesangial cell (Figure 2–16, FSA–11). It is phagocytic and morphologically similar to muscle cells.

Filtration Barrier. The term *filtration* implies that the bulk flow of solvent through a porous barrier carries with it molecules or particles sufficiently small to pass through the barrier. The driving force for the filtration process is the net pressure difference across the barrier. The filtration rate of a given molecular species is proportional to the pressure difference across the barrier and the barrier's conductance or ease of solute passage through it. The glomerulus behaves as an ultrafilter which passes electrolytes and small organic molecules like glucose, but largely retains plasma protein and larger elements. In the case of albumin the retention is not complete. The concentration of albumin in Bowman's space is about 0.1 per cent of that in plasma. From this fact, it is inferred that the effective pore size of the filtration barrier is near the molecular size of albumin (70,000).

The filtration barrier is far from an homogeneous entity; it consists of a series of complex structures which collectively determine the kinds of particles which enter Bowman's space. For a molecule to enter Bowman's space from the glomerular circulation, it must first traverse the capillary endothelium. It appears that this structure presents little impediment to filtration, because large molecules (450,000) move through

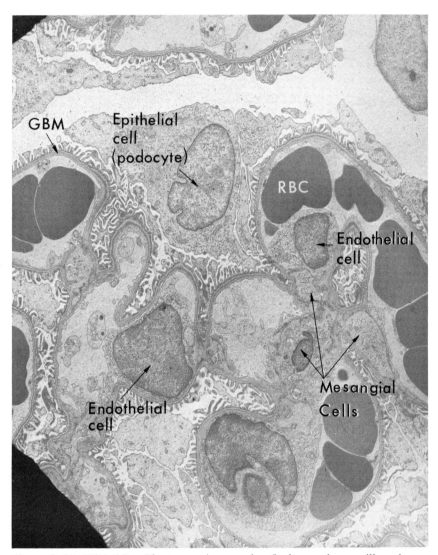

Figure 2–16 (FSA–11). Electron micrograph of glomerular capillary loops, showing relationship between epithelial cells, endothelial cells, and mesangial cells.

the endothelial pores, which are larger and more irregular than in other fenestrated capillaries. There is some disagreement about whether these pores are bridged by a thin layer of material like that seen in fenestrated capillaries in other regions of the body. The next obstacle encountered is the basement membrane. Tracer studies have failed to reveal the presence of discrete pores like those of the capillary endothelium. Nevertheless, the matrix of this collagen-like structure must be sufficiently loose to permit molecules of the size of myeloperoxidase (MW 160,000) or smaller to pass freely. The final obstacle is the pedicel layer of the podocytes, bridged by the filtration slit membrane (Figure 2–17, FSA–12). This filtration slit membrane appears to offer a significant resistance to the passage of high molecular weight substances into Bowman's space, but molecules of horseradish peroxidase (MW 40,000) appear to pass through readily.

Filtration Pressure.   In man the approximate mean hydrostatic pressure (mm Hg) is 100 in the renal artery, 90 in the glomerular capillaries, and 15 in Bowman's space (Figure 2–18). The plasma protein osmotic (oncotic) pressure within the glomerulus is about 30 mm Hg; it is essentially zero in Bowman's space. Since the glomerular capillary hy-

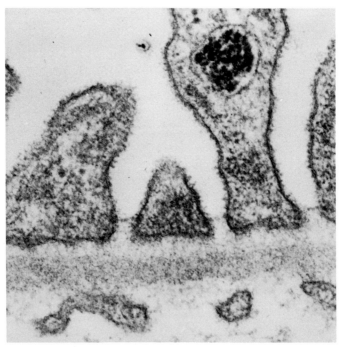

Figure 2–17 (FSA–12).   High-power electron micrograph of the filtration barrier, showing podocytes with filtration slit membranes, glomerular basement membranes, and pores of the endothelial cells.

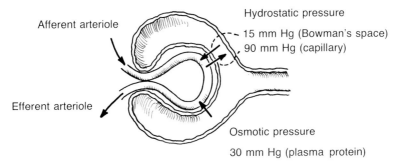

Figure 2–18. Glomerular filtration pressure.

drostatic pressure is opposed by the osmotic pressure, the pressure gradient driving filtration is equal to (90 − 15) − (30 − 0) or 45 mm Hg. Table 2–1 lists some factors that cause abnormal filtration.

The Concept of "Clearance" and the Measurement of GFR. In a limited sense, one of the functions of the kidney is to excrete or "clear" solutes from the blood. A measure of this "clearance" function is the volume of plasma per unit time (typically, ml/min) which is completely cleared of a solute. Obviously, this is an apparent and not an actual volume. No single milliliter of blood has all of its solute removed in one transit through the kidney; rather, a little solute is removed from each of the many milliliters of blood perfusing the kidneys. Although it is possible to measure the "clearance" of any solute which is excreted by the kidney, the clearance of a substance which is only filtered and is not transported by the tubular cells has special merit because its measurement will represent the GFR.

The concept of clearance is not difficult, but an understanding of the equation used in its calculation comes somewhat more slowly. The following example will help to illustrate the mathematical relationships

Table 2–1. Factors influencing glomerular filtration.

A. Changes in permeability caused by renal disease
B. Changes in hydrostatic pressure
    1. In the glomerular capillaries
        a. Drop in systemic arterial pressure below 90 mm Hg no longer stabilized by autoregulation
    2. In Bowman's capsule
        a. Ureteral obstruction
        b. Edema of kidney inside tight renal capsule
C. Changes in osmotic pressure
    1. Change in oncotic pressure of plasma proteins, as in hypoproteinemia
D. Change in the number of nephrons
    1. Disease destroying glomeruli
    2. Loss of renal tissue through trauma or surgery

involved in its formulation. Consider substance "X" which could be used to measure GFR because it is freely filtered but not reabsorbed or secreted by tubular cells. The symbolic relationships discussed concerning "X" are represented as follows:

$$[X]_u = \text{concentration of "X" in urine}$$

$$[X]_p = \text{concentration of "X" in plasma}$$

$$\dot{V} = \text{urine flow rate}$$

$$GFR = \text{glomerular filtration rate}$$

$$\dot{V}[X]_u = \text{quantity of "X" excreted in urine}$$

$$GFR[X]_p = \text{quantity of "X" filtered by glomeruli}$$

In the steady state, as much of "X" leaves the nephron each minute as is filtered through the glomeruli, or

$$\dot{V}[X]_u = GFR[X]_p$$

Thus, knowledge of the urinary excretion rate and plasma concentration of "X" are sufficient to allow computation of the GFR. For example, if 250 mg/min of "X" is being excreted, the same amount has entered the nephrons. If the plasma concentration is 2 mg/ml, then 125 ml/min of glomerular filtrate was produced to account for the quantity excreted:

$$GFR = \frac{[X]_u \, \dot{V}}{[X]_p} = \frac{250 \text{ mg/min}}{2 \text{ mg/ml}} = 125 \text{ ml/min}$$

Several materials, like the "X" used above, are suitable for the estimation of filtration rate. The measurement of GFR is important for an understanding of renal diseases and for the quantitative assessment of tubular transport. It is, therefore, desirable to have a convenient and quantitative method of estimation. This can be done by measuring the renal clearance of certain specific solutes. The classic solute which is used for measurement is inulin, a fructose polymer having a molecular weight of 5,000 and a diameter of 15 Å; it is not bound to plasma or tissue protein. The principal disadvantage of inulin is that it must be continuously infused to maintain constant plasma levels. The normal GFR is considered to be 70 ml/min/m², or approximately 120 ml/min for an average-sized adult with a surface area of 1.73 m².

A comparison of the renal clearance of any solute with that of inulin or some other comparable marker of GFR will give information as to possible solute transport by the renal tubules. For example, a substance which is not protein bound and is freely filterable but has a clearance less than that of inulin has undergone net tubular reabsorption, whereas a substance with a clearance greater than that of inulin has obviously been secreted by tubular cells. Certain substances like p-aminohippurate (PAH) are rapidly secreted by tubular cells and are almost entirely "cleared" from the blood perfusing the kidneys. Thus, substances such as PAH will measure the total effective renal blood flow to functional nephrons.

In clinical practice the clearance of endogenous creatinine is often used as an estimate of GFR. Creatinine is an end-product of creatine phosphate catabolism, and its plasma concentration and total renal excretion are reasonably constant. In contrast to urea, its plasma concentration is little influenced by dietary changes. Unfortunately, it suffers the disadvantage of some tubular secretion and does not give a true measure of GFR. Despite this defect, the creatinine clearance is convenient and adequate for most clinical purposes.

Reflection on the clearance equation will reveal several interesting concepts which have important clinical implications. These can best be illustrated by reference to the endogenous creatinine clearance. If, in the steady state, it is accepted that the urinary excretion of creatinine is constant, then an inverse proportionality is seen between the creatinine clearance and the plasma concentration of creatinine.

$$C_{creat} = \frac{\dot{V}\,[creat]_u}{[creat]_p}$$

Such a relationship is illustrated in Table 2–2, where the inverse but proportional changes in the plasma creatinine and creatinine clearances are seen *when creatinine excretion is constant.*

Clinically, this information is useful in determining changes in renal function (GFR) through single measurements of plasma creatinine concentration. For example, a patient with an initial creatinine clearance of 100 ml/min and a creatinine plasma concentration of 1 mg/100 ml has a urinary excretion rate of creatinine of 1000 μg/min or 1.4 gm daily. If, on a later date, the serum creatinine concentration has risen to 5 mg/100 ml due to loss of functioning nephrons and it is assumed that the total

Table 2–2.

C_{creat} ml/min	$\dot{V}[creat]_u$ μg/min	$[creat]_p$ mg/100 ml
100	100	1
50	100	2
20	100	5
10	100	10
5	100	20

urinary excretion of creatinine has remained constant, then it is clear that the creatinine clearance is one-fifth of the previous value, or 20 ml/min. With increasing renal disease, this precise relationship begins to fail as creatinine metabolism increases in the gut flora and total urinary excretion falls. However, the relationship is good enough to serve as a tool for following most patients with progressive renal dysfunction. The following diagram may help to illustrate the previously described concepts relating GFR changes to those of serum creatinine and urea concentration (Figure 2–19).

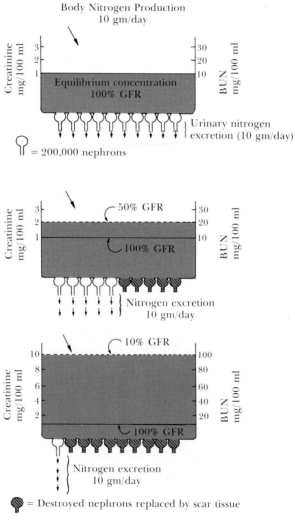

Figure 2–19. Typical increase in plasma creatinine and BUN with decreasing GFR when body production of urea and creatinine remains constant.

Proximal Convoluted Tubule

General. A filtration rate of 120 ml/min (about 180 L/day) in an adult would soon deplete the body of water and solutes unless a large fraction of the filtrate was reabsorbed. Of the 120 ml of filtrate formed per minute in the glomeruli, approximately 119 ml are reabsorbed as the fluid passes through the various segments of the nephrons and collecting ducts, leaving only 1 ml to be excreted as urine. The bulk of this filtrate is reabsorbed by the proximal tubule. About 60 to 80 per cent of the filtered water and electrolytes and essentially all of the filtered glucose, amino acids, and protein are removed in this segment. The proximal tubule also participates in plasma detoxification by secreting many exogenous organic acids and bases into its lumen.

Structure. The structure of the proximal tubule is well suited to its task of transport. The proximal tubules of kidneys perfused with either blood or histological fixatives have open lumens, while tissues fixed without perfusion, such as renal biopsies, have collapsed tubules. Evidently, tubular pressures are equal to or greater than interstitial pressures during perfusion. Because the proximal tubule is the longest part of the nephron, it is seen more frequently in histological sections than other nephron segments found in the cortex. The proximal convoluted tubular cells are very complex in shape, with numerous lateral interdigitating processes which serve to increase the amount of lateral cell membranes and lateral intercellular space (Figure 2–20, FSA–13).

The cytoplasm of the cells is highly acidophilic; the nuclei lie basally. The luminal margin of the cells is lined by a *brush border layer* which consists of finger-like extensions of the plasma membrane called *microvilli* (Figure 2–21, FSA–14; Figure 2–22, FSA–15), similar to those of the small intestine. The microvilli of the intestinal epithelium have been shown to participate in sugar and amino acid absorption, and the similarity between transport properties in these two tissues strongly suggests that the transport processes are the same for the kidney.

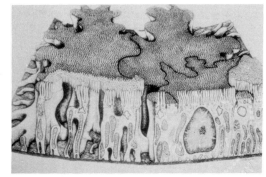

Figure 2–20 (FSA–13). Relationships between proximal tubule cells. (From Bulger, R., Amer. J. Anat. *116*:237–256, 1965.)

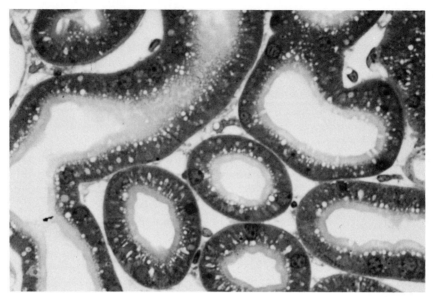

Figure 2-21 (FSA-14). Low-power photomicrograph of proximal tubule. The pale-staining brush border can be seen on the luminal aspect of each proximal tubule.

By electron microscopy, mitochondria are seen to lie in large interdigitating processes of adjacent cells (Figure 2-23, FSA-16). The interdigitating processes, by increasing the lateral surface area of the epithelium, enhance the exchange of solutes and water between tubular cells and peritubular capillaries. The cell membranes of these lateral processes may be more than passively involved in transport. The presence of the mitochondria, together with histochemical evidence of ATPase activity of the membrane, support the view that an active pump is located in these lateral membranes.

General Characteristics of Tubular Transport. One of the principal activities of the renal tubules is to transport solutes and water across tubular cells. Such transport is termed *reabsorption* when its direction is from the tubular lumen to the interstitial fluid and *secretion* when its direction is from the interstitial fluid to the tubular lumen. In the case of tubular secretion, amounts of solute greater than those filtered appear in the urine.

Quantitatively, the net tubular transport (T_X) of a substance "X" is the difference between the amount filtered (GFR $\times$ X_p) and the amount excreted (V $\times$ X_u). Symbolically, this is represented as:

$$T_X = (GFR \times [X]_p) - (\dot{V} \times [X]_u)$$

A positive T_X indicates tubular reabsorption, and a negative T_X indicates secretion.

Transport always depends upon an energy supply. It is convenient to classify tubular transport according to the source of the energy which is utilized in the transfer process. The process is termed *active transport* if the substance moves against a gradient of electrical potential or chemical concentration. If the substance, on the other hand, migrates down an electrochemical gradient, the process is termed *passive transport* or *diffusion*. Table 2–3 contains a list of commonly transported substances classified into "active" or "passive" categories.

Theoretically, any active transport process has quantitative limits. Most active renal transport falls into two general categories: (1) those associated with a transport maximum (Tm), and (2) those showing a limitation in the gradient developed between interstitium and tubular lumen. Substances showing Tm-limited characteristics are: glucose, amino acids,

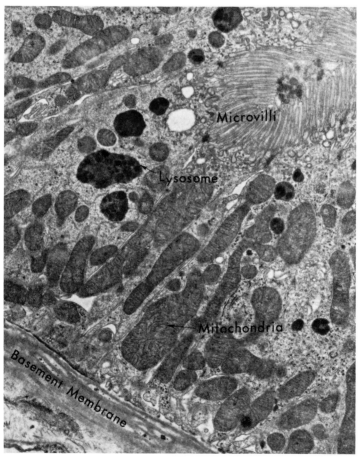

Figure 2–22 (FSA–15).   Electron micrograph of proximal tubule. Brush border at upper right and basement membrane at lower left. Note elongated mitochondria.

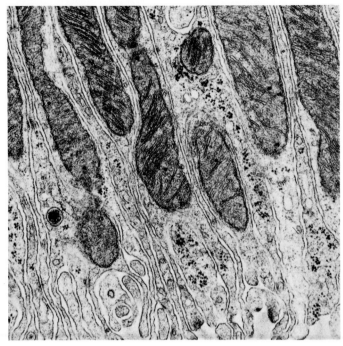

Figure 2–23 (FSA–16). High-power electron micrograph of a proximal tubular cell, demonstrating complex interdigitation of adjacent cells.

phosphate, sulfate, and organic acids. The gradient-limited pattern is seen in the transport of sodium and hydrogen.

Glucose Reabsorption. The reabsorptive mechanism for glucose illustrates well the characteristics of an active Tm-limited reabsorptive

Table 2–3. Types of Renal Tubular Transport

ACTIVE		PASSIVE	
Reabsorption	*Secretion*	*Reabsorption*	*Secretion*
Sodium	Hydrogen	(produced by solute reabsorption)	
Potassium	Potassium	Water	None
Calcium	Ammonium	Chloride	
Magnesium	Certain organic	Acetone	
Phosphate	bases	Ethanol	
Sulfate	Certain organic	CO_2	
Glucose	acids	Urea	
Amino acids	Creatinine	(influenced by urinary pH difference)	
Urate		Bicarbonate	Ammonium
Protein		Weak acids in	Weak acids in
		acid urine	alkaline urine
		Weak bases in	Weak bases in
		alkaline urine	acid urine

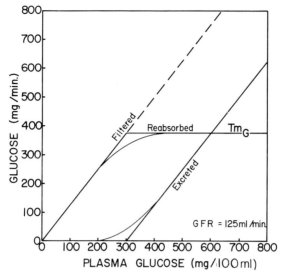

Figure 2–24. Determination of the renal threshold for glucose in man. (From *Physiology of the Kidney and Body Fluids* by Robert F. Pitts. Copyright © 1968 by Year Book Medical Publishers. Used by permission.)

transport system. With normal plasma glucose levels (90 to 100 mg/100 ml) and GFR (120 ml/min), the filtered glucose presented to the proximal tubules is completely reabsorbed. Glucose begins to appear in the urine when the filtered load approaches 216 mg/min/m², the approximate Tm for glucose. Glucose filtered in excess of Tm is excreted in the urine. The higher the plasma concentration of glucose, the greater is the quantity excreted.

It has been found that over a wide range of plasma glucose concentration, a constant rate of glucose reabsorption is present. This quantity represents the maximum tubular reabsorptive capacity for glucose and is shown in Figure 2–24.

Because tubular reabsorption is complete when the plasma concentration of glucose is normal, there is no excretion of glucose and the glucose clearance is nil. As the plasma glucose concentration increases and the maximum tubular reabsorptive capacity is exceeded, glucose appears in the urine and the clearance becomes measurable. The higher the plasma glucose concentration, the greater is the clearance, and at very high concentrations the glucose clearance approaches the GFR (Figure 2–25).

Certain active transport mechanisms, such as those concerned with glucose, may be involved in the transfer of two or more substances. For example, xylose, fructose, galactose, and glucose are apparently reabsorbed by a single transport mechanism, although their affinity for transport varies considerably. If the plasma glucose concentration is

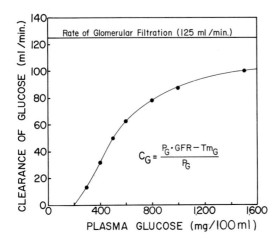

Figure 2-25. Clearance of glucose as a function of plasma concentration of glucose. (From *Physiology of the Kidney and Body Fluids* by Robert F. Pitts. Copyright © 1968 by Year Book Medical Publishers. Used by permission.)

raised to a level sufficient to saturate the glucose reabsorptive mechanism, reabsorption of xylose is completely blocked and the clearance of xylose becomes equal to GFR. Contrariwise, if plasma xylose concentration is elevated there is no appreciable interference with the reabsorption of glucose, as the affinity of glucose for transport far exceeds that of xylose.

Amino Acid Reabsorption.   At least three active transport processes have been distinguished: (1) for a group of basic amino acids including cystine, lysine, ornithine, and possibly arginine; (2) for an acid group including glutamic and aspartic acids; and (3) for a neutral group which includes the remainder. This classification is based primarily on studies of competition for transport by similar molecules. However, the observation that patients with cystinuria (an inborn error of transport) also excrete ornithine, arginine, and lysine but not other amino acids further supports this classification.

The rate of reabsorption at high plasma levels of all amino acids has not been studied. However, with the exception of histidine, most exhibit a Tm. The overwhelming preference for reabsorption of the naturally occurring L-isomers further demonstrates the specificity of these processes.

Renal reabsorption does not normally play a role in the regulation of plasma glucose or amino acid concentrations because reabsorptive maxima for these substances are poised well above the usual filtered loads. Plasma levels of these substances are normally determined by exchange with their intracellular pools.

Reabsorption of Endogenous Organic Anions.   A number of naturally occurring organic anions are excreted in the urine in small amounts. Although net tubular reabsorption can be demonstrated, their transport characteristics are obscured by multiple factors: secretion and reabsorption, metabolism by the tubule cells, high passive permeabilities, transport by other segments of the nephron, transport rates dependent on acid-base balance, or all of these. This group includes: citrate, malate, β-hydroxybutyrate, ascorbic acid, and urate.

Secretion of Organic Acids and Bases. Exogenous organic bases, such as tetraethylammonium (TEA), and exogenous organic acids, such as *p*-aminohippurate (PAH) and penicillin, are rapidly excreted once they enter the circulation. In addition to being filtered, they are actively transported (secreted) into the tubular fluid. Most of the acids compete with each other for secretion, as do most of the bases. However, competition between acids and bases is not observed. The secretory processes also exhibit transport maxima; therefore, at high plasma levels filtration may become the dominant mode of excretion. Some of these substances, for example PAH, are so avidly secreted that at plasma levels well below saturation, they are completely cleared from the renal plasma.

The characteristics of the secretory mechanism which transports PAH and other compounds of this class are illustrated in Figure 2–26. Over a range of plasma concentration from 1 to 10 mg/100 ml, the rates of excretion, secretion, and filtration increase in proportion to the increase in plasma level. Above 10 mg/100 ml, secretion of PAH becomes constant and independent of plasma concentration. The maximum rate of secretory transport of PAH averages 46 mg/min/m². If the plasma concentration of PAH is <60 mg/100 ml, tubular secretion ac-

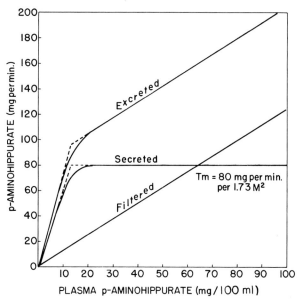

Figure 2–26. Rates of filtration, secretion, and excretion of PAH as functions of plasma concentration. (From *Physiology of the Kidney and Body Fluids* by Robert F. Pitts. Copyright © 1968 by Year Book Medical Publishers. Used by permission.)

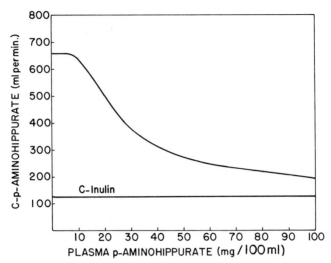

Figure 2–27.   Clearance of PAH as a function of plasma concentration. (From *Physiology of the Kidney and Body Fluids* by Robert F. Pitts. Copyright © 1968 by Year Book Medical Publishers. Used by permission.)

counts for the major fraction of excreted PAH, whereas if plasma concentration exceeds this concentration, filtration accounts for the major excreted fraction. Because of these characteristics, the clearance of PAH asymptotically approaches the GFR at high plasma concentrations as the contribution of secretion becomes negligible (Figure 2–27).

Because of the avidity with which PAH is secreted at plasma levels well below transport saturation, it almost completely clears from the renal plasma in a single circulation through the kidney, and the concentration in the renal vein is small. Consequently, the clearance of PAH at low plasma levels (<10 mg/100 ml) is a measure of renal blood flow. This is sometimes called effective renal blood flow, because PAH in the renal vein is not truly absent; some non-cortical and perirenal regions drain into this vessel.

Sodium and Water.   By the end of the proximal tubule, reabsorption of Na^+ and water reduces the volume of filtrate to 20 to 40 per cent of its initial value. Osmotic gradients between peritubular capillaries and proximal tubular fluid are never observed; therefore, both must remain isosmotic with arterial plasma throughout proximal tubular reabsorption. Since Na^+ and associated anions (Cl^- or HCO_3^-) account for most of the osmotic activity of proximal tubular fluid, and water for its volume, it follows that Na^+ and water are simultaneously reabsorbed and that their ratio is set by plasma osmolality. Present evidence indicates that *water reabsorption is passive* and coupled to *active Na^+ reabsorption.*

The observation that renal oxygen consumption parallels Na^+ reabsorption is in accord with this concept of active Na^+ transport.

Unlike Tm-limited reabsorption, proximal tubular reabsorption of sodium chloride is *not* saturable but does appear to exhibit gradient-limited characteristics. A central issue in the renal regulation of Na^+ excretion is the interdependence which exists between tubular reabsorption and glomerular filtration. Under a variety of circumstances, the fraction of the glomerular filtrate reabsorbed in the proximal segment is *relatively* constant in the face of varying rates of filtration, a state often referred to as *glomerulotubular balance.* Although relatively independent of changes in filtration, the fractional reabsorption of Na^+ in the proximal tubule is influenced by certain extrarenal factors (the extracellular volume) as well as intrarenal factors (pressure, volume).

Potassium Reabsorption. The reabsorption of Na^+ and water tends to concentrate other constituents of the filtrate relative to their peritubular plasma concentration and thereby promotes their passive reabsorption. This effect alone, however, is insufficient to account for the total reabsorption of potassium, which is about 90 per cent complete by the end of the proximal tubule. Therefore, it is necessary to postulate that *potassium reabsorption is active.*

Anion Reabsorption. Both chloride and bicarbonate reabsorption are probably passive, although the evidence does not allow a clear decision. The reabsorption of bicarbonate, which plays a pivotal role in acid-base balance, is influenced by many factors which are discussed in greater detail in a subsequent section.

The polyvalent anions, phosphate and sulfate, like sodium, are actively reabsorbed; but unlike sodium, their transport mechanisms are saturable (Tm type). The Tm of these processes are set at the normal filtered load (about 0.11 and 0.07 mMols/min respectively); therefore, an increase in plasma concentration causes the filtered loads to exceed their Tm and, as a result, phosphate and sulfate are excreted in the urine. Correspondingly, if the plasma levels of phosphate and sulfate drop, the filtered load falls below Tm and they are conserved; thus, the proximal tubular transport mechanisms serve to regulate the plasma levels of these ions. Futher regulation of plasma phosphate is achieved through parathyroid hormone. An increase in the concentration of this hormone decreases the Tm for phosphate.

Urea Reabsorption. Urea, like water, is reabsorbed passively in both the proximal and distal nephron. These substances flux between lumen and interstitial fluid down osmotic and concentration gradients. Urea is the primary waste product of protein catabolism and is found in significant quantities in plasma, especially in persons on high-protein diets. The plasma concentration of urea (measured as blood urea nitrogen and abbreviated to BUN) is dependent not only upon

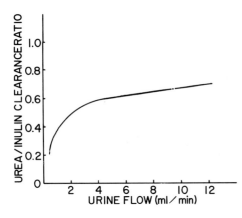

Figure 2–28. Variation of urea/ inulin clearance ratio with urine flow in man. (From *Physiology of the Kidney and Body Fluids* by Robert F. Pitts. Copyright © 1968 by Year Book Medical Publishers. Used by permission.)

renal excretion, but also on its production from protein catabolism and metabolism by gut bacteria. Clinically, the plasma concentration of urea is frequently elevated due to marked catabolism, even though renal function is not impaired. In order to distinguish an increased production of urea as the cause of BUN elevation in contrast to renal causes, it is useful to inspect the ratio of BUN to serum creatinine. Ordinarily this ratio is no greater than 15:1. Ratios which exceed this value are usually associated with excessive catabolism.

In contrast to previously discussed substances, the clearance of urea is variable, depending upon the urine flow rate (Figure 2–28). When the urine flow exceeds 2 ml/min, the average clearance of urea is 40 ml/min/m². Since the normal GFR exceeds this value, it is evident that urea is being reabsorbed. This dependency of urea clearance on flow rate, as well as the observation that urea clearance is independent of plasma concentration, suggests that urea reabsorption is passive. Micropuncture studies have shown that a large fraction (70 to 80 per cent) of filtered urea is reabsorbed during the normal antidiuretic state because of its high tubular permeability and the progressive reabsorption of water.

Protein Reabsorption.   Although small amounts of plasma proteins (mainly albumin) do penetrate the glomerular filtration barrier, virtually none is found in the final urine because it is largely reabsorbed by the proximal tubule. The cells of the proximal convoluted tubule are characterized by the presence of a highly specialized apparatus for the uptake of protein. Between the bases of the microvilli, tubular invaginations appear which are capable of picking up filtered proteins (Figure 2–29, FSA–17). These proteins appear to be transported into the lysosomes and are broken down. At the present time, little is known about the transport of intact proteins across any cell layer, including that of the proximal convoluted tubule.

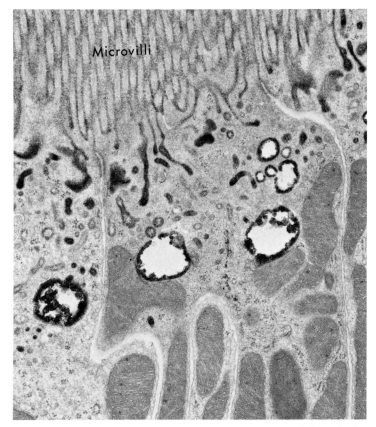

Figure 2–29 (FSA–17). High-power electron micrograph of the apical portion of a proximal tubule. The dark material is horseradish peroxidase entering small canaliculi between microvilli and finally collecting in vacuoles immediately above the mitochondria.

Loop of Henle

Structure. The loop of Henle consists of the descending thick limb (or straight part of the proximal tubule), the thin limb (in all but the most cortical nephrons) and the ascending thick limb (or straight part of the distal tubule).

Descending Thick Limb (Figure 2–30, FSA–18). As the proximal convoluted tubule enters into the medullary ray to begin the loop of Henle, the morphology of the tubule changes slightly. Cells from the descending thick limb (or straight part of the proximal tubule) tend to be more cuboidal than those of the convoluted portion. The brush border is still well developed.

Thin Limb (Figure 2–31, FSA–19; Figure 2–32, FSA–20). The loop of Henle courses toward the tip of the renal papilla and then turns

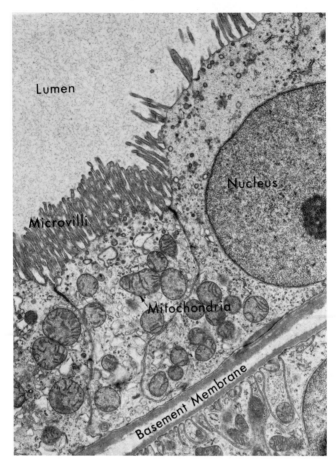

Figure 2–30 (FSA–18). Electron micrograph of descending thick limb. Note cell interdigitations and rounded mitochondria.

back, forming a hairpin loop. The loop can have an extremely short or absent thin limb section in cortical nephrons or a longer thin limb section in juxtamedullary nephrons. The thin limb is best distinguished from other segments on the basis of its low, flattened epithelium. However, even these thin cells frequently have interdigitating processes. The cells are of greater height near their nuclei. Mitochondria are small and infrequently seen in these cells.

Ascending Thick Limb (Figure 2–33, FSA–21; Figure 2–34, FSA–22). These tubules are similar in appearance to the distal convoluted tubules. The nucleus lies in an apical position in these cells and the basal cytoplasm is filled with elongate, closely packed mitochondria in interdigitating compartments. Only a few microvilli are found along the apical surface.

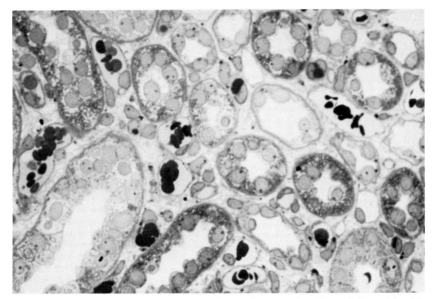

Figure 2–31 (FSA–19). Low-power photomicrograph of medulla with thin limb, capillaries, and collecting ducts.

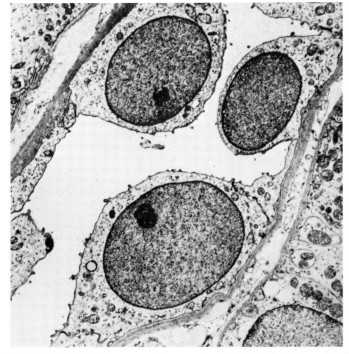

Figure 2–32 (FSA–20). Electron micrograph of thin limb. The epithelial cells are low-lying, containing few cell organelles and few basilar interdigitations.

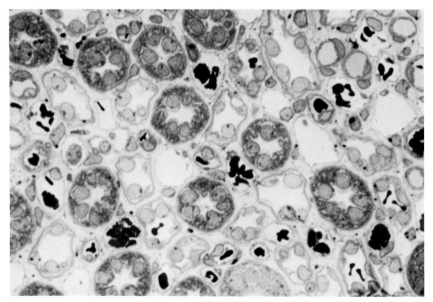

Figure 2–33 (FSA–21).   Photomicrograph of ascending thick limb.

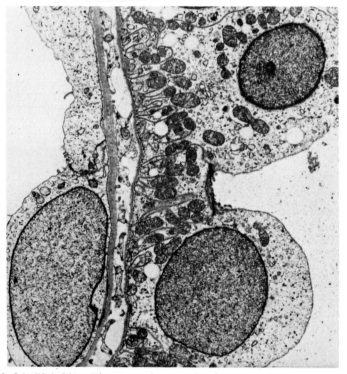

Figure 2–34 (FSA–22).   Electron micrograph of an ascending thick limb on the right and a thin limb on the left.

Distal Convoluted Tubules

Structure. The ascending thick limb returns to the cortical region in the medullary ray and then proceeds to pass between the afferent and efferent arterioles of its glomerulus and continues on as a distal convoluted segment. In the region where the distal tubule lies near the arterioles, the distal tubular cells are modified to form the macula densa (discussed below). The epithelial cells lining the distal convoluted tubule are lower in height and frequently have a smaller diameter than those in the proximal convoluted tubules. More nuclei are seen in a cross-section of a tubule (Figure 2–35, FSA–23; Figure 2–36, FSA–24). The cytoplasm of the cells is less eosinophilic than those of the proximal tubule. The cells do not possess a brush border. The mitochondria are again in the interdigitating processes, which extend laterally from the cell border. As the distal convoluted tubule is shorter than the proximal convoluted tubule, fewer cross-sections of the distal convoluted tubule are seen in histological sections of cortex.

Collecting Duct

Structure. The distal convoluted tubule empties into the collecting duct. The collecting duct courses through the cortex into the medullary

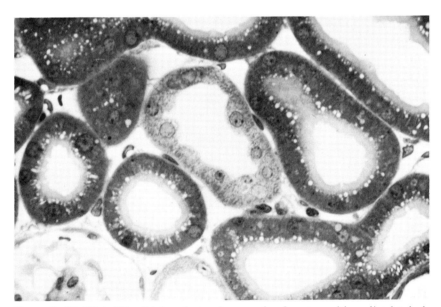

Figure 2–35 (FSA–23). Light photomicrograph of cortex with a distal tubule among proximal tubular profiles.

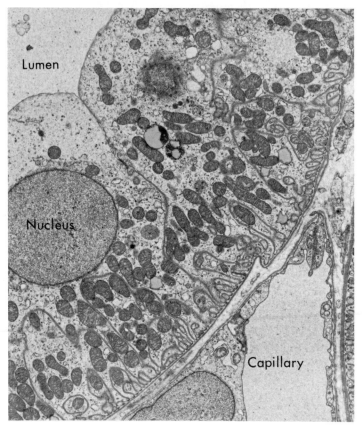

Figure 2-36 (FSA-24). Electron micrograph of the mid-region of the distal tubule.

ray, and through the medulla to empty into the pelvis. In the cortex the collecting duct cells (Figure 2-37, FSA-25; Figure 2-38, FSA-26) are cuboidal in shape. The collecting tubules consist of two types of cells, the principal (or light cells) and the intercalated (or dark cells) (Figure 2-39, FSA-27). The principal cells have relatively clear cytoplasm with well-defined cell margins, centrally placed nuclei, and multiple, small, randomly oriented mitochondria. The intercalated cells are much less common and are absent in the inner medullary portion. The intercalated cells have more intensely staining cytoplasmic matrix and larger, more numerous mitochondria. The cells increase in height as the collecting ducts penetrate into the medulla and course toward the pelvis, where the cells are frequently columnar (Figure 2-40, FSA-28).

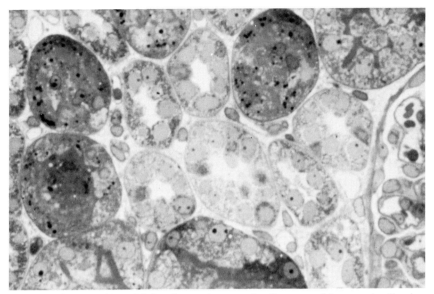

Figure 2-37 (FSA-25).   Light photomicrograph of cortex with several collecting ducts in the middle of the field.

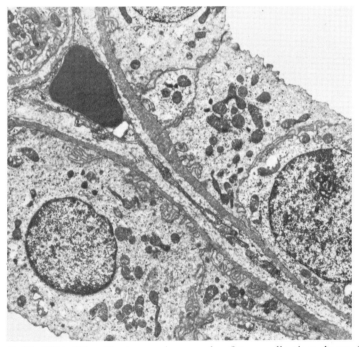

Figure 2-38 (FSA-26).   Electron micrograph of two collecting ducts. Brush border, lateral interdigitations, and cell organelles are sparse.

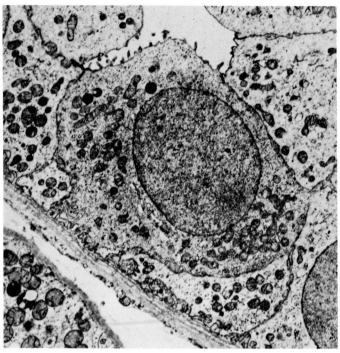

Figure 2-39 (FSA-27).   Electron micrograph of a distal tubule, showing a dark cell with numerous rounded mitochondria and other cell organelles. (From Myers, C. E., Bulger, R. E., Tisher, C. C., and Trump, B. F., Laboratory Investigation *15*:1921–1950, 1966.)

Transport Properties of the Nephron Distal to the Proximal Tubule

Concentration and Dilution of Urine.   Man can, according to his needs, conserve water by producing a concentrated urine or eliminate excess water by producing a dilute urine. The kidney accomplishes this by a mechanism involving a countercurrent multiplier (the loop of Henle) and countercurrent exchangers (the looping capillaries (Figure 2–41, FSA–29) and the collecting duct). The osmolality of the interstitial fluid in the outer medulla and papilla, unlike the cortex, is hyperosmotic to arterial plasma. This osmolality, which may reach 1200 mOsm/Kg at the papilla, arises from the countercurrent multiplication produced by the trapping of sodium ions in the medulla. These ions are actively transported into the interstitium by the ascending limb of the long loops of Henle. The presence of a hypertonic medulla allows the extraction of water from collecting duct fluid as it flows through the papilla. Whether or not enough water is extracted to produce a concentrated urine depends on the water permeability of the collecting duct (controlled by the level of circulating antidiuretic hormone), the rate of urine flow and the amount and type of solute reaching this site.

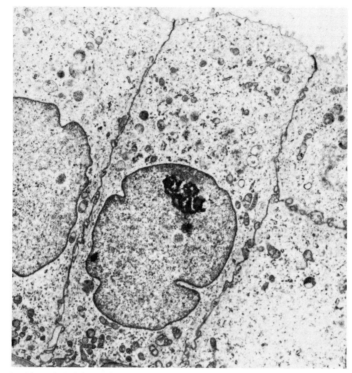

Figure 2–40 (FSA–28). Electron micrograph of collecting duct near tip of papilla, with projections showing columnar appearance.

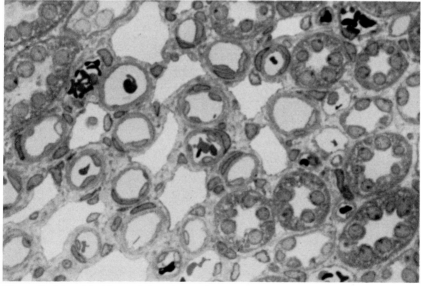

Figure 2–41 (FSA–29). Light photomicrograph of a bundle of arterioles (vasa rectae) with multiple capillary spaces between adjacent tubules.

Operation of the Countercurrent Mechanism (Figure 2–42)

Hypertonic Medulla. Consider a small volume of 300 mOsm/kg fluid filtered across the glomerulus. As it flows through the proximal tubule, absorption of Na^+ and water greatly reduces its volume without changing its osmolality (still 300 mOsm/kg). However, upon entering the descending limb of Henle's loop, its osmolality begins to increase and continues to do so until by the tip of the loop, or the region of the papilla, its osmolality is 1200 mOsm/kg, or about four times that of plasma. During the return passage through the ascending limb, this same element of fluid undergoes a reversal in osmolality. However, a net decrease in osmolality occurs so that fluid entering the distal tubule is hypotonic (100 mOsm/kg) to proximal tubular fluid (300 mOsm/kg).

The existence of an osmotic gradient from the outer medullary junction to the papilla rests on sound experimental observations; however, the tubular mechanisms which generate the medullary gradient are not clearly understood. Theoretically, the gradient might arise as follows. As the small volume of fluid flows through the ascending limb, Na^+ is actively pumped out of the tubular lumen. Because the ascending limb is impermeable to water (heavy lines in Figure 2–42), water does not follow the Na^+ and the fluid becomes hypotonic relative to the fluid volume in the apex of the papilla. The sodium ions pumped into the interstitium raise its osmolality, causing water to leave the water-permeable descending limb (thin lines in Figure 2–42). Thus, as a volume of

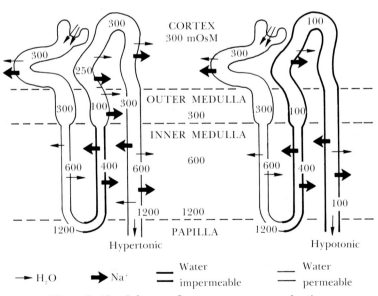

Figure 2–42. Schema of countercurrent mechanism.

tubular fluid descends the loop, it becomes progressively more concentrated, so that fluid which started out at 300 mOsm/kg at the outer medullary junction becomes 1200 mOsm/kg at the tip of the loop, only to fall to 100 mOsm/kg as it leaves the ascending limb. Urine dilution in the ascending limb is accomplished without an increase in volume by a continued removal of solute (mainly Na^+ and attendant anions) without transport of water. The poor water permeability exhibited by the ascending limb is characteristic of this segment and is not influenced by extra-renal factors such as antidiuretic hormone (ADH). At any given level, the osmolality of the descending limb exceeds that of the ascending limb by only a few hundred mOsm/kg; the large gradient along the loop arises from the progressive transport of Na^+ from ascending limb fluid by a low intensity pump.

Water moves passively across the distal nephron just as in the proximal tubule. But water permeability of the distal nephron is variable, unlike that of the proximal tubule, which is constant. The water permeability of the distal nephron varies with the circulating level of antidiuretic hormone (ADH).

Production of Hypertonic Urine. In the presence of a high ADH titer, the distal tubule and collecting duct become highly permeable to water. Consequently, hypotonic fluid (100 mOsm/kg) entering the distal tubule rapidly loses water until it becomes isotonic with the surrounding cortical interstitium (300 mOsm/kg). As this fluid flows through the medullary collecting ducts, it continues to lose water to the hypertonic medullary interstitium and emerges from the collecting duct hypertonic to cortical or arterial plasma.

Production of Hypotonic Urine. When ADH titer is low, distal nephron permeability to water is low. Thus, hypotonic fluid (100 mOsm/kg) passing through the distal nephron loses very little water. The exact dilution of the final urine depends also on the amount of sodium reabsorbed by the distal nephron. As one might expect, the most dilute urines are produced by water-loaded and sodium-depleted individuals.

Sodium Reabsorption. Sodium transport in the ascending limb of Henle's loop and the distal nephron differs from that of the proximal tubule in its capacity to reabsorb sodium against large gradients (ratio of sodium concentration in tubular fluid:plasma of 1:1000). It is influenced by aldosterone, with an increase in hormone titer increasing the distal nephron transport capacity.

Although the proximal tubule is responsible for recovering most of the sodium in the glomerular filtrate, a small fraction always reaches the distal nephron. Thus, the distal nephron serves as the final arbiter of sodium elimination. Under normal conditions, the distal nephron transport is set to nearly match the fraction of the filtered load which is not reabsorbed in the proximal tubule, and an amount of sodium is excreted which will maintain sodium balance. This excreted amount is approximately equal to that ingested in the diet. Similarly, during sodium loading or deprivation, appropriate adjustments are made to either eliminate or reabsorb the necessary sodium to maintain balance. How these adjustments are made has been an area of intense investigation, but a clear explanation is not yet available. It does seem likely that changes in sodium balance produce proportional changes in the fractional reabsorption of sodium in the proximal tubule. Thus, with sodium loading, less sodium is reabsorbed by the proximal tubule and a larger load is delivered to the distal nephron; this is not completely reabsorbed, so that the increment in glomerular filtrate delivered out of the proximal tubule now appears as final urine. This less complete reabsorption by the distal nephron may be due to an absolute inhibition of the transport mechanism mediated by sodium loading and an expansion of the extracellular volume. Alternately, at these high rates of delivery, the increased excretion of sodium may simply reflect a distal transport mechanism operating beyond the normal saturation limit. As previously mentioned, more or less of the sodium load reaching the distal nephron may be reabsorbed by raising or lowering the transport with changes in aldosterone titer which, in turn, are closely connected to body sodium content.

Potassium Secretion. The distal transport of potassium is quite variable; however, potassium excretion ranges around 20 per cent of the glomerular filtration rate. Some years ago, it was observed that in patients with chronic renal disease and a markedly reduced GFR, the clearance of potassium frequently exceeded the inulin clearance, suggesting tubular secretion. Since that time, many experiments have been done which clearly demonstrate the capacity of the kidney to secrete potassium. In view of the many micropuncture studies which have clearly shown that the proximal tubule reabsorbs more than 90 per cent of the filtered potassium, the distal nephron must secrete potassium. Further studies have confirmed this conclusion and shown the distal convoluted tubule as the site of secretion. The rate of potassium secretion appears to depend on the intracellular concentration of potassium in this site and the electrochemical gradients developed. Thus, the plasma potassium concentration, potassium balance, acid-base status, sodium balance, and aldosterone all influence potassium secretion. The direction of these changes can be seen in Table 2–4.

Hydrogen Ion Excretion. The renal regulation of acid-base balance is related to its capacity to control the concentration of extracellular bicarbonate and secrete hydrogen ion against an electrochemical gradient. During its transit from the glomerulus to the papilla, the tubular fluid is modified in two ways which permit the formation of an acid urine. First, bicarbonate is reabsorbed from the tubular fluid; and second, hydrogen ions are added to the tubular fluid, forming a urine with a low pH.

Because bicarbonate is reabsorbed at a slightly more rapid rate than

Table 2-4. Factors Affecting Potassium Secretion.

ACID-BASE	
Resp. alkalosis	↑
Met. alkalosis	↑
Resp. acidosis	↓
Met. acidosis	↓
FLUID-ELECTROLYTE BALANCE	
Sodium loading	↑
Sodium deprivation	↓
Potassium loading	↑
Potassium depletion	↓
Water loading	—
DRUGS	
Acetazolamide (met. acid. & alkaluria)	↑
Thiazide	↑
Mannitol or urea diuresis	↑
Aldosterone	↑
Spironolactone	↓
Triamterene	↓

↑ Increase
↓ Decrease
— No change

chloride, the concentration of bicarbonate in samples of proximal fluid diminishes gradually along the nephron from about 25 mEq/L at the beginning to about 10 to 15 mEq/L at the end. By the end of the proximal tubule, about 80 to 90 percent of the filtered bicarbonate has been reabsorbed, with a reduction in the tubular fluid pH to approximately 6.5 to 7.0. In the loop of Henle and the distal tubule, bicarbonate reabsorption continues keeping pace with the reabsorption of water or slightly exceeding it, so that the pH of the tubular fluid in this part of the nephron is 6.0 to 6.5. In the collecting duct, the pH of the tubular fluid falls to that of the final urine. Acidification in the distal nephron results from a process of hydrogen ion secretion (H^+) which can generate a hydrogen ion gradient of over 1000:1, a value which reflects a blood pH of 7.4 to a urine pH of 4.4. As noted below, such active secretion of hydrogen ions is important in the excretion of hydrogen ions in combination with bases such as phosphate and ammonia.

Hydrogen ions excreted by the kidney appear in the urine in three chemical forms: (1) free hydrogen ions, (2) ammonium, and (3) titratable acid. Free hydrogen ions are present in very small quantities and are responsible for determining the urine pH, which can vary between about 4.0 and 8.0. Although these pH values represent minute amounts of hydrogen ion, the urine pH is of great importance in determining the total amount of hydrogen ion excreted. Ammonia (NH_3) produced in the kidney, or elsewhere in the body, binds with hydrogen ion to form ammonium ion (NH_4^+), which accounts under normal circumstances for about 60% of the net hydrogen ion excretion. The remaining 40% of metabolic hydrogen ions is excreted as titratable acid. This term is used to describe hydrogen ions bound to weak acid anions, which are measured by titrating the urine with sodium hydroxide back to the pH of the blood. The total excretion of hydrogen ions in these forms amounts to 60 to 100 mEq daily, but in no way gives insight into the actual capacity for hydrogen ion excretion. In a quantitative sense, the daily reabsorption of approximately 5100 mEq of bicarbonate in exchange for a comparable secretion of hydrogen ions is of greater significance. Therefore, an understanding of bicarbonate reabsorption is of paramount importance in discussing renal acidification and body acid-base balance.

Bicarbonate Reabsorption. Under normal circumstances, the rate of bicarbonate reabsorption is carefully adjusted to maintain a constant plasma bicarbonate concentration around 25 mEq/L. Elevations above this level lead to a prompt excretion of alkaline urine with a high bicarbonate concentration. In many ways, the process of bicarbonate reabsorption resembles a Tm limited mechanism in which increases in filtered load above the Tm lead to loss of the excess bicarbonate in the urine. But in fact, no true Tm for bicarbonate is demonstrable, and the rate of reabsorption can be altered by several physiologic influences of which the following are the most important:

1. *Carbon dioxide tension* (P_{CO_2}): An increase in body P_{CO_2} raises the rate of bicarbonate reabsorption and, conversely, a decrease in the P_{CO_2} lowers bicarbonate reabsorption.

2. *Chloride balance:* When body chloride is selectively depleted, bicarbonate reabsorption increases. Expansion of the extracellular space with sodium chloride decreases bicarbonate reabsorption.

3. *Carbonic anhydrase:* Inhibition of this enzyme by certain drugs exerts a powerful inhibitory effect on bicarbonate reabsorption and results in a large diuresis of bicarbonate, a rise in urine pH, and a metabolic acidosis.

This latter observation strongly suggests that carbonic anhydrase

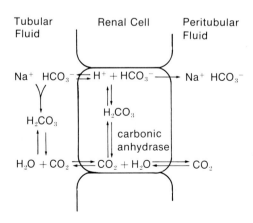

Figure 2–43. Model of bicarbonate reabsorption.

plays a critical role in the mechanism for bicarbonate reabsorption. The most widely held concept of the mechanism for bicarbonate reabsorption is shown in Figure 2–43. Carbonic anhydrase within the cells of the tubules catalyzes the hydration of carbon dioxide to carbonic acid, which dissociates into H^+ and HCO_3^-. The bicarbonate ion generated by this reaction moves out of the cell along an electrochemical gradient and back into the extracellular fluid. The hydrogen ion which is left behind is secreted into the tubular fluid, where it reacts with a filtered bicarbonate ion, reforming carbonic acid and then carbon dioxide and water (this latter reaction is also believed to be catalyzed by carbonic anhydrase in the brush border of the proximal tubule). The carbon dioxide diffuses back into the cell, completing the cycle. Thus, filtered bicarbonate is transferred out of the tubular fluid in the form of carbon dioxide. Carbonic anhydrase inhibitors interfere with this sequence by inhibiting the hydration reaction and thus, the generation of hydrogen ions from CO_2 and water in the cell. This limits the amount of hydrogen ion available for secretion into the tubule. Conversely, an increase in P_{CO_2} increases the rate of carbonic acid formation in the cell, providing more hydrogen ions for secretion. Therefore, according to this theory, the effects of both carbonic anhydrase inhibitors and P_{CO_2} on bicarbonate reabsorption are attributed to their influence on the rate of generation of intracellular hydrogen ions.

Ammonium Excretion.   The weak acid, ammonium, and its conjugate base, ammonia, constitute an acid-base pair which reacts according to the equation:

$$NH_3 + H^+ \rightleftarrows NH_4^+$$

Ammonia is uncharged and lipid soluble; it penetrates cell membranes readily and, hence, diffuses swiftly to all parts of the kidney. It reacts with hydrogen ions in each of the different fluid compartments of the kidney, forming ammonium ions, NH_4^+ (Figure 2–44). The quantity of NH_4^+ formed in a particular compartment will depend on (1) the pH of the fluid in that compartment and (2) the partial pressure of ammonia in the kidney. When the pressure of ammonia is constant, differences in pH between collecting duct fluid and renal venous blood determine the distribution of NH_4^+ between these two compartments and thus regulate the proportion of NH_4^+ leaving the kidney by these routes. That is, when the pH of collecting duct fluid is low (pH<6), creating a large difference in pH between renal venous blood and urine, NH_4^+ excretion in the urine will be high. When collecting duct (and hence, urine) pH rises, NH_4^+ will be shifted, by means of NH_3 diffusion, from urine to renal venous blood, decreasing NH_4^+ excretion. Thus, changes in urine pH regulate the distribution of NH_4^+ between urine and renal venous blood, providing an important mechanism for adjusting the rate of NH_4^+

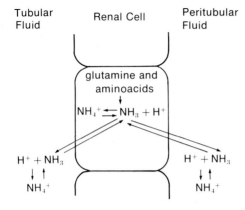

Figure 2–44. Model of ammonium excretion.

excretion in the urine. The passive, physical chemical process responsible for this behavior is termed *"nonionic diffusion"* (Figure 2–45).

The second important factor determining ammonium excretion, the pressure of ammonia, depends on (1) the rate of entrance of ammonium in the renal arterial blood, which is usually relatively constant, and (2) the rate of synthesis of ammonia in the kidney. Large amounts of ammonia are synthesized in renal tissue from the amino acid glutamine.

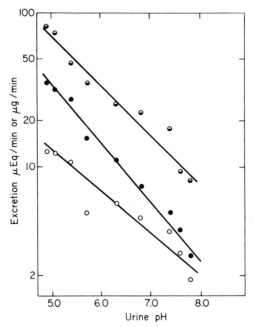

Figure 2–45. Relation of ammonium excretion to urinary pH. (From Orloff, J., and Berliner, R. W., Journal of Clinical Investigation, *35*:223–235, 1956.)

Changes in systemic acid-base balance regulate the rate of ammonia formation from glutamine in the kidney, metabolic acidosis stimulating ammonia production and metabolic alkalosis inhibiting it. This alteration in the rate of ammonia formation, and hence in NH_4^+ excretion, in response to changes in acid-base balance represents one of the most important mechanisms by which the kidney can adjust H^+ excretion in response to changing rates of H^+ production.

Titratable Acid. When hydrogen ions are secreted into the tubular lumen causing the pH of the tubular fluid to fall, anions of weak acids bind hydrogen ions. This reaction can be written:

$$A^- + H^+ \rightleftarrows HA$$

where A^- is the anion of any weak acid HA.

The following factors determine the rate of titratable acid excretion:

1. *The quantity of buffer anion:* Over the pH range of urine, phosphate is the major buffer which contributes to the formation of titratable acid. Hence, the amount of titratable acid excreted varies in proportion to the amount of phosphate excreted. The amount of phosphate excreted per day is primarily determined by the composition of the diet.

2. *Acid strength of the buffer:* A buffer with pK (negative logarithm of the dissociation constant) midway between the pH of blood and that of the final urine will bind maximum amounts of H^+ per millimole of buffer. Phosphate has a pK which enables it to form large amounts of titratable acid in moderately acid urine.

3. *Urine pH:* Within the physiologic pH range, phosphate exists almost entirely in two forms, $HPO_4^=$ and $H_2PO_4^-$ and the relative proportion of these ions present in any solution is determined by the pH. As hydrogen ions are added to the tubular fluid, decreasing its pH, some of the $HPO_4^=$ will be converted to $H_2PO_4^-$ and this quantity of H^+ will be

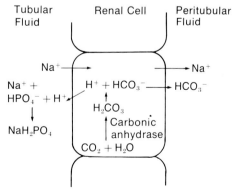

Figure 2–46. Model of titratable acid excretion.

measured as titratable acid. When urine pH is 5.0 or less, creatinine and urate also bind hydrogen ions in significant amounts and contribute to the titratable acid measured (Figure 2–46).

The Regulation of Urine pH.   As previously indicated, urine pH is a major factor in determining the excretion of ammonium and titratable acid. Unfortunately, the mechanisms regulating urine pH are poorly understood. Some of the more important factors influencing urine pH are:

1. *The amount of tubular fluid bicarbonate delivered to the collecting duct:* If large amounts of bicarbonate are present in the tubular fluid when it arrives in the collecting duct, secreted H^+ will be neutralized by reacting with bicarbonate, forming CO_2 and H_2O, and urine pH will be high. Consequently, variations in proximal bicarbonate reabsorption may be reflected by variation in urine pH.

2. *Poorly reabsorbable anions:* If a high proportion of the chloride in the tubular filtrate is replaced by sulfate, phosphate, or other poorly reabsorbed anions, the pH of the urine will fall. Such poorly reabsorbable anions increase the electrochemical potential across the tubule and thereby stimulate H^+ secretion.

3. *Interrelationship between Na^+, H^+, and K^+ transport in the distal nephron:* In order to maintain a normal electrochemical gradient in the distal nephron, each hydrogen ion secreted must be accompanied by reabsorption of some other cation or secretion of an anion. No evidence for significant anion secretion has been found. Since sodium is the principal cation reabsorbed in the nephron, hydrogen ion secretion is generally viewed as being associated with sodium reabsorption. For example, administration of aldosterone stimulates sodium reabsorption and hydrogen ion secretion, causing urine pH to fall. Under certain circumstances, a reciprocal relationship appears to exist between the concentration of hydrogen ions in the urine and the state of potassium balance. Thus, in potassium chloride depletion an acid urine is secreted; conversely, administration of potassium salts leads to a more alkaline urine. These relationships between H^+ secretion and sodium and potassium excretion are not obligatory, and numerous exceptions to them can be found.

4. *Systemic acid-base balance:* A temporary fall in urine pH accompanies induction of systemic acidosis; if the acidosis persists, the urine pH rises again toward normal. A commonly used test of the ability of the kidney to secrete hydrogen ions depends on this relationship.

The Juxtaglomerular Apparatus (JGA)

Structure.   The JGA (Figure 2–47, FSA–30; Figure 2–48, FSA–31) consists of four portions: (1) a specialized portion of the afferent arteriole containing characteristic granulated cells; (2) a portion of the distal tubule lying between the straight portion of the distal tubule and the

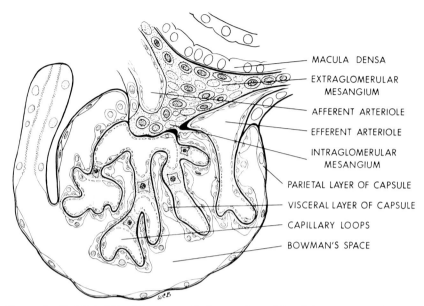

MACULA DENSA

EXTRAGLOMERULAR
MESANGIUM

AFFERENT ARTERIOLE

EFFERENT ARTERIOLE

INTRAGLOMERULAR
MESANGIUM

PARIETAL LAYER OF CAPSULE

VISCERAL LAYER OF CAPSULE

CAPILLARY LOOPS

BOWMAN'S SPACE

Figure 2–47 (FSA–30). Diagram of glomerulus with JGA. (From Bulger, R., *in* Histology, 3rd edition, edited by R. O. Greep and L. Weiss. McGraw-Hill Book Co., New York, 1973.)

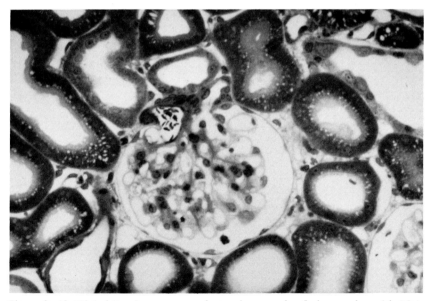

Figure 2–48 (FSA–31). Low-power photomicrograph of glomerulus with JGA. Red blood cells are in afferent arteriole.

convoluted portion of the tubule, called the macula densa; (3) a cushion
of cells at the vascular pole of the glomerulus that are continuous with
the mesangium, termed the extraglomerular mesangium; and (4) a
region of the efferent arteriole.

Near the vascular pole, the smooth muscle cells of the media of the
afferent arteriole are found to contain characteristic granules which can
be identified by their staining properties and morphology; they are
thought to contain renin. It is thought that the granulated cells represent modified smooth muscle cells from the arteriolar media. Granulated cells have also been seen in the wall of the efferent arteriole which
lies adjacent to the macula densa.

The Macula Densa.   The macula densa (or dense spot) consists of
cells forming the wall of the distal tubule in the region where the ascending limb returns to the glomerulus of its origin (Figure 2–49, FSA–32).
The tubule runs between the afferent and efferent arterioles in this
region. The term "dense spot" is derived from the fact that the cell
nuclei are close together in this region, forming what looks like a dense
spot in hematoxylin and eosin sections. In the region of the macula
densa, distal tubular cells have a different morphology. The nuclei lie
closer to each other, the Golgi apparatus is located in the basal region of

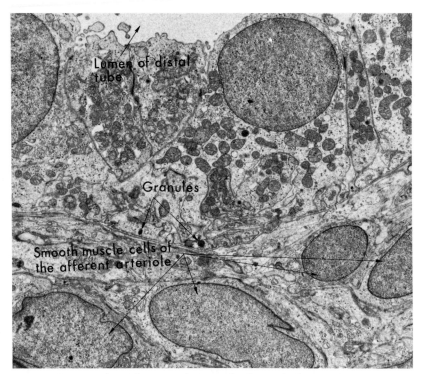

Figure 2–49 (FSA–32).   Electron micrograph of macula densa cells with complex
basilar interdigitations and dark granules at base.

the cell instead of the apical region, and the interdigitating processes in the basal cytoplasm are oriented laterally. It appears that these cells are morphologically polarized with their active surface toward the base instead of the apex as in the adjacent distal tubular cells.

Function of the JGA. Although our understanding is incomplete, it is clear that the JGA is involved in *volume* and *pressure* regulation. The integrative way in which extracellular volume and blood pressure are controlled will be discussed in Chapter 3. The discussion here will concern basic mechanisms which may operate within the JGA to produce this physiological control. Much evidence has accumulated that renin is formed in the granules of the JGA cells. Renin is a proteolytic enzyme which catalyzes the conversion of a plasma protein to angiotensin I. This substance is cleaved by a converting enzyme, mainly in the lung, to the potent octapeptide, angiotensin II, which then stimulates the release of aldosterone by the zona glomerulosa of the adrenal cortex. Although angiotensin is also a potent vasoconstrictor, its effect on blood pressure control is probably mediated more through its effect in controlling sodium regulation via aldosterone secretion than through a direct vasoconstrictor effect.

The specific signals perceived by the JGA to secrete renin are still unknown. Two theories are currently in vogue. According to the baroreceptor hypothesis, the renal afferent arterioles and JG cells respond to changes in stretch which could be secondary to changes in vascular volume and pressure. The alternate theory conceives the macula densa as a primary sensing element in the renin release mechanism. It is postulated that a decrease in sodium reabsorption by the macula densa cells results in renin release. Available evidence has also indicated the importance of the renal sympathetic nerve and various humoral agents including sodium and potassium ions, angiotensin, and the catecholamines in releasing renin. A plausible working hypothesis is that both receptors are operative but the extent of dominance varies with the physiological or pathophysiological conditions. The proposed pathway for the control of renin release is seen below.

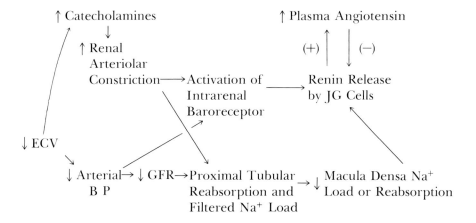

Recently, it has been suggested that renal autoregulation and glomerulotubular balance may be a consequence of an intrarenal regulation through the JGA. A central requirement of this theory is the ability of the JGA to form vasoactive angiotensin II locally. There is now experimental evidence that renin, renin substrate, and converting enzyme activity are all present at the juxtaglomerular site. The incorporation of a tubulovascular feedback mechanism for the autoregulation of glomerular filtrate would imply that some characteristic of tubular fluid at the macula densa produces a variable amount of angiotensin locally, which acts as a controller of glomerular filtrate rate. Experiments have suggested that the intratubular sodium concentration in the macula densa segment or reabsorption by the cells in this area could be the adequate stimulus for the control of GFR. Autoregulation of blood flow may only be a by-product of this sodium load-adjusting mechanism.

Renal Interstitium

The interstitium is scarce in the cortex but more abundant in the medulla. Here the interstitium contains a population of elongate interstitial cells (Figure 2–50, FSA–33). These cells are oriented with their long axes perpendicular to the long axes of the tubules and vessels. The function of these cells is at present unknown, although crude extracts of tissue containing large numbers of interstitial cells possess vasodepressor substances.

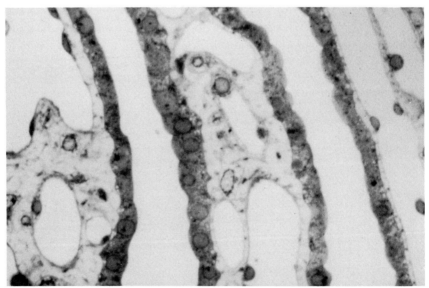

Figure 2–50 (FSA–33). Light photomicrograph of medulla with multiple interstitial cells.

THE URINARY COLLECTING AND VOIDING SYSTEM

The urinary conducting system is made up of a group of connected ducts and reservoirs lined with transitional epithelium. Their walls contain smooth muscle that actively propels urine from the renal collecting tubules to the bladder and out of the body. While there is a flow of ions and substances across the cells lining this system, the net exchange is small under normal circumstances.

Renal Pelvis and Ureter. The urinary conducting system begins at the renal papilla. Under the mucosa of the papilla is a circular layer of smooth muscle which contracts intermittently to propel urine from the papillary ducts into the renal pelvis (Figure 2–51, FSA–34). This may change tissue pressure within the papilla itself. The renal pelvis is basically a funnel which in turn empties into the upper ureter. Contractions of the circularly arranged muscle in the wall of the pelvis are seen by cineradiography to move towards the ureter. Pressures within the main body of the pelvis remain low during these contractions, but pressures as high as 40 mm Hg may occur low in the funnel (near the ureter) during periods of high flow, such as occur in response to diuretics.

Ureter Anatomy and Relationships. The ureters are flattened fibromuscular tubes about 25 to 29 cm in length, extending between the renal pelvis and the urinary bladder (Figure 2–1; Figure 2–52, FSA–35). They consist of two portions, the abdominal ureter superiorly and the

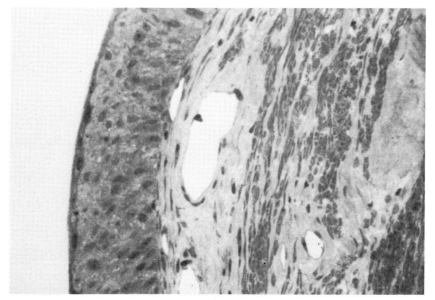

Figure 2–51 (FSA–34). Photomicrograph of calyceal region of kidney, showing transitional epithelium and adjacent smooth muscle fibers. (From Bulger, R., *in* Histology, 3rd edition, edited by R. O. Greep and L. Weiss. McGraw-Hill Book Co., New York, 1973.)

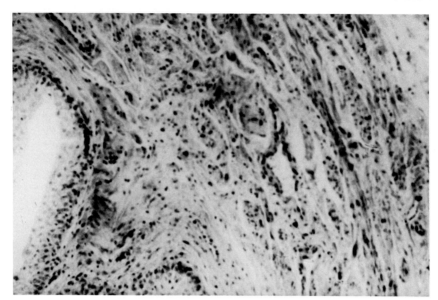

Figure 2–52 (FSA–35).   Light photomicrograph of ureter, showing transitional epithelium on the left and multiple layers of smooth muscle.

pelvic ureter inferiorly. The abdominal ureter is in the retroperitoneal space where it courses down the anterior surface of the psoas muscle almost parallel with the median line but inclining slightly medially. It crosses the brim of the bony pelvis at the bifurcation of the common iliac artery. Each ureter is crossed obliquely by the testicular or ovarian vessels. The right ureter is also crossed anteriorly by the right colic and ileocolic vessels; the left ureter, by the left colic vessels. The arteries of the abdominal portion of the ureter are branches of the renal artery and of the testicular or ovarian artery. The pelvic ureter continues caudally in a retroperitoneal position along the lateral wall of the bony pelvic cavity. The pelvic portion of the ureter receives branches of the superior vesical artery of the internal iliac system. At the level of the ischial spine the pelvic ureter bends medially and anteriorly to enter the bladder wall, through which it passes in an oblique fashion and terminates in a slit-like meatus at the lateral angle of the trigone. When the bladder is distended, the upper and lower walls of the ureter are pressed together, which prevents reflux of urine from the bladder into the ureter. Reflux is considered abnormal. There are three normal areas of slight ureteral narrowing where renal stones may lodge: the ureteropelvic segment, the bony pelvic brim, and the ureterovesical junction.

The arterial blood supply to the ureter is received from both ends. The proximal ureter receives branches from the renal artery. The distal end receives branches from the internal spermatic, hypogastric, and inferior vesical arteries, creating possible collateral channels if localized arterial obstructions occur.

The urine is moved down the ureter by peristaltic waves of contraction propagated through the smooth muscle. An extensive network of nerve fibers has been demonstrated among the smooth muscle cells of the urinary tract, but their function in regard to the peristaltic waves is not clear. No definite pacemaker has been found in the renal pelvis or ureter, but it has been shown that a ureter that is completely cut and reanastomosed does not resume normal contractions across the anastomosis for a period of about four weeks. This suggests that either intact nerves or contiguous cell membranes are needed for propagation.

Each of the peristaltic waves carries only about five percent of the urine in the pelvis down to the bladder. Distention of the renal pelvis and ureter increases the frequency of contraction, the normal response to an increase in the flow of urine. As the rate of flow of urine increases further, ureteral contraction waves continue to increase in amplitude until the whole ureter remains open between contraction waves. Patients with diabetes insipidus may produce 10 to 20 liters of urine per day and their ureters are often completely open on urography.

Acute distention of the ureter is caused by an elevation in the resting pressure and the associated increased rate of ureteral contraction. However, in chronic distention, resting pressure and rate of peristalsis may be normal. Even when the ureter is distended, peristaltic waves can still move fluid from the kidney to the bladder. During such waves, which do not close the ureteral lumen completely, urine in the middle of the channel moves toward the bladder while urine adjacent to the ureteral wall actually travels in the opposite direction. Although the net flow is towards the bladder, the reverse flow of urine near the wall may carry bacteria from the bladder to the kidney.

Distention of the ureter results not only in an increase in diameter but also in an increase in length. Since the ureter is relatively fixed at the ureteropelvic junction and at the bladder, the increase in length associated with distention causes tortuosity in the course of the ureter.

Bladder Structure and Relationships. The urinary bladder acts as a reservoir for urine. It contracts periodically during micturition to void its contents to the outside through the urethra. It varies in size and configuration according to the degree of filling. In the infant it is an abdominal organ, but in an adult it lies in the true bony pelvis. When considerably distended, its dome may rise out of the pelvis toward the umbilicus. Superiorly the bladder is covered by the peritoneum. Anteriorly it abuts the symphysis pubis. Posteriorly it is separated from the rectum in the male by the ampulla of the vas and the seminal vesicles and in the female by the uterus and vagina. The floor of the bladder, called the trigone, is bounded by the two ureteral orifices and the bladder neck.

The bladder is lined by a layer of transitional epithelium supported by a loosely textured submucosal layer which allows the transitional cell mucosa to be thrown into folds or rugae when the bladder is empty. Outside the submucosal layer is an intertwining network of smooth muscle fibers (the detrusor muscle), which is continuous down through the bladder neck into the urethra. In the proximal urethra the fibers form a poorly defined structure called the internal sphincter. In the male, the urethra extends through the prostate (prostatic urethra) and is anchored there solidly relative to the bony pelvis by the musculofascial urogenital diaphragm (the membranous urethra) (Figure 2–53, FSA–36). This is the only solidly fixed portion of the lower urinary tract near the bladder, a fact which becomes important in trauma when the relatively mobile bladder may be torn loose from its moorings at the membranous urethra and the urethra ruptured. In the urogenital diaphragm there are striated muscle fibers oriented in such a way as to form an external sphincter surrounding the membranous urethra at the apex of the prostate in the male and the distal one-third of the urethra in the female. This sphincter may be relaxed voluntarily, but its principal function is to prevent leakage of urine from the bladder during episodes when intra-abdominal pressure increases (as occurs during coughing or

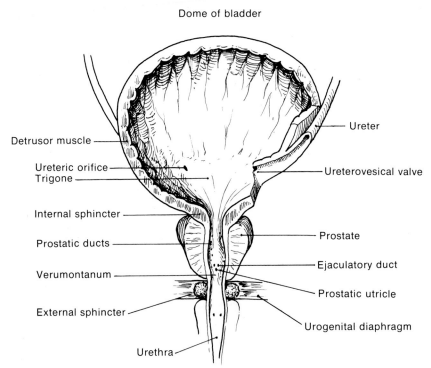

Dome of bladder

Detrusor muscle

Ureteric orifice
Trigone

Internal sphincter

Prostatic ducts

Verumontanum

External sphincter

Urethra

Ureter

Ureterovesical valve

Prostate

Ejaculatory duct

Prostatic utricle

Urogenital diaphragm

Figure 2–53 (FSA–36). Urinary bladder, showing prostate and intramural ureter.

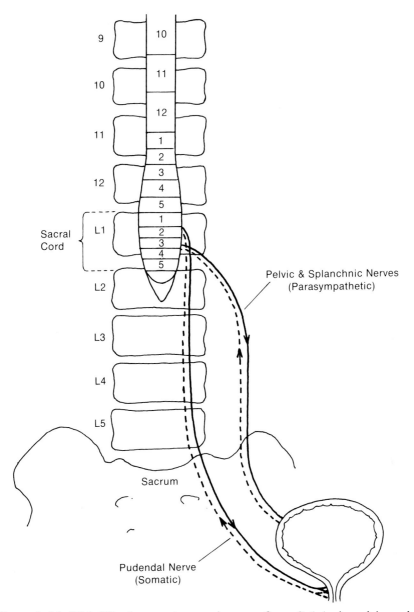

Figure 2-54 (FSA-37). Innervation to detrusor from S 1-4 via pelvic and splanchnic nerves, and to external sphincter via pudendal nerves.

sneezing). It may be voluntarily contracted in order to stop voiding and is normally relaxed upon initiation of micturition. It apparently does not play a part in maintaining continence in the normal resting state, which is done in the region of the internal sphincter.

The blood supply of the bladder is provided by the superior and middle vesical arteries arising from the umbilical branch of the internal iliac artery. Smaller branches also arise from the common trunk of the internal pudendal and inferior vesical arteries and in the female from the uterine and vaginal arteries.

The abundant lymphatics of the bladder drain primarily to external iliac nodes and partially to the internal and common iliac nodes. This is significant, since bladder tumors spread mostly via the lymphatics.

The nerve supply to the detrusor is from the sacral region (S_2 to S_4) of the parasympathetic system (Figure 2–54, FSA–37). The external sphincter receives somatic (voluntary) supply via the pudendal nerve (S_2 to S_4).

Sensory nerves are also segmented in the S_2-S_4 area. The bladder reflex arc is then below L_5 and receives only cortical control above that level.

Micturition. Because the bladder functions as a reservoir, urine may be disposed of at convenient intervals. Resting pressure during storage is low (10 cm H_2O) and emptying is normally complete upon micturition. The normal bladder is able to expand to accommodate fairly large quantities of urine (400 to 600 cc) without raising the pressure above 20 cm of water.

When the bladder is distended by filling there is a small initial rise in pressure to 5 to 10 cm of water. The bladder then accommodates to fur-ther increases in volume with very little rise in pressure until micturition is initiated. As the detrusor contracts, the intravesical pressure increases to 20 to 40 cm H_2O. At the same time the longitudinal fibers in the trigone contract to open the bladder neck, and the external sphincter voluntarily relaxes to allow voiding.

It should be remembered that the sacral portion of the spinal cord is at the level of T_{10-12} and that trauma to the spinal column in this region or below may interrupt the reflex arc of the bladder, while above this region they will interrupt the central control of micturition. The intactness of the nerve supply to the bladder can be checked by checking other reflex arcs that use similar pathways (the bulbocavernosus reflex, or the anal wink). Sensory changes in S_1-S_4 distribution (the perineum and perineal region) should be noted.

Prostate Gland Anatomy and Relationships. The prostate gland is the largest accessory sex gland of the male, and its function is to contribute to the production of the seminal fluid. It is a firm elastic gland weighing approximately 20 gm and having the shape of a truncated cone. It lies immediately below the bladder and surrounds the prostatic urethra. The conical apex rests upon the deep layer of the urogenital diaphragm. The ejaculatory ducts pass through the gland posteriorly to enter the urethra. The prostate is surrounded by a network of thin-walled veins (the prostatic plexus) which connects with the prevertebral veins and numerous perforating veins draining the bony pelvis. During sudden increased intra-abdominal pressure the vertebral venous system serves as a shunt for blood returning to the heart from the lower extremities. The connections of this plexus also account for the metastatic spread of tumors to the vertebra, which may occur in cancer of the prostate.

The prostate gland is of clinical importance because of its propensity for hyperplasia and neoplasia, which affects 30 per cent of all males over 50 years of age.

The prostatic urethra of the male contains the first fusiform dilatation in the course of the urethra. The floor of the prostatic urethra is deformed by a slight elevation called the colliculus seminalis (verumontanum) through which the ejaculatory ducts enter the urethra. The membranous urethra is contained in the urogenital diaphragm and is surrounded by the external urethral sphincter. The anterior urethra consists of three parts: (1) the bulbous, (2) the pendulous or penile, and (3) the glandular part. The bulbous urethra is the proximal portion of the anterior urethra immediately below the urogenital diaphragm. It is a fusiform dilatation of the urethra into which open the ducts of the bulbo-urethral (Cowper's) glands. The pendulous urethra is of uniform caliber and traverses the external penis to the glans. Here it becomes the glandular urethra, containing a third area of fusiform dilatation, and opens to the surface through the external urethral meatus.

The female urethra is a short tubular structure approximately 3.5 cm in length, lying between the symphysis pubis and the lower portion of the anterior vaginal wall. The muscular coats are continuous with those of the bladder, and the entire length of the urethra and bladder neck area function together as a sphincter mechanism.

Chapter 3

HORMONES, DRUGS, AND THE KIDNEY

Some drugs have been appropriately called "wonder-drugs" inasmuch as one wonders what they will do next.

SAMUEL E. STUMPF (1918–   )

The principles of renal handling of solutes, metabolites, and water have been outlined in the previous chapter. To a large degree, these functions are carried out as intrinsic properties of the cells constituting the kidney. In addition to this *intrinsic* regulation, renal function is constantly being modified by natural *extrinsic* factors such as hormones. Such hormonal influences are not entirely from extrarenal sources, as the kidney produces at least one hormone (renin) which is active in producing extrarenal and probably intrarenal effects on tubular transport. In addition, quite apart from its effects on fluid and electrolyte balance, the kidney also has been shown to be involved in the hormonal stimulation of erythropoiesis. Thus, anemia often accompanies renal failure; erythrocytosis, on occasion, occurs with hypernephroma or hydronephrosis.

As knowledge of renal physiology has increased, clinical pharmacologists have felt inclined to manipulate renal function by administering chemical compounds which produce potent changes in transport mechanisms. Such capabilities can be useful in certain disease states, but, like a two-edged sword, can produce problems of their own which may be worse than the disease for which they were given.

This chapter will discuss hormones produced by the kidney as well as those altering its function. In addition, commonly used drugs which affect or are affected by a change in renal function will be discussed.

HORMONES PRODUCED BY THE KIDNEY

Renal Erythropoietic Factor (REF). The REF-erythropoietin system, like that of the renin-angiotensin system, is composed of a renal fac-

70

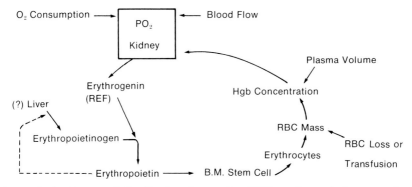

Figure 3–1. Proposed feedback schema for REF-erythropoietin control of red cell production. Dotted line indicates possible inhibition of erythropoietinogen by erythropoietin. Changes in RBC mass and hematocrit also influence schema.

tor (REF or erythrogenin) acting on a plasma substrate to produce an active end product. The operation of this system is diagrammed in Figure 3–1.

The exact anatomic location of cells producing REF has not been established. Damage to either tubules or glomeruli interfere with the production of erythropoietin. Normal red cell production is stimulated by erythropoietin which, in turn, is sensitive to slight changes in renal oxygen supply and tissue needs. Experimentally, it has been possible to increase erythropoietin output by (1) a reduction in renal blood flow, (2) the production of increased intrarenal pressure through ureteral obstruction, and (3) microinfarction of the kidney. Clinical expressions of these mechanisms, although uncommon, have been described in man.

The primary site of erythropoietin action is thought to be a hemopoietic stem cell. It is claimed that erythropoietin may also produce an increase in the absolute number of normoblasts in the bone marrow, stimulate hemoglobin synthesis in existing normoblasts, and cause release of marrow reticulocytes.

Renin. This proteolytic enzyme is apparently derived from the granules contained in JG cells. Its physiological role in regulating angiotensin and aldosterone has been previously described (Chapter 2).

HORMONES AFFECTING RENAL FUNCTION

Antidiuretic Hormone. ADH or vasopressin is synthesized by the hypothalamus and stored in the posterior pituitary. Under normal conditions it is released by osmotic or volume stimuli and is active in the kidney only in producing an enhancement of water permeability in the distal nephron, with a resultant conservation of water and a production of hypertonic urine.

Aldosterone. Following the demonstration of an abnormality in renal tubular reabsorption of sodium by adrenalectomized animals, a tremendous volume of evidence has accumulated indicating that aldosterone is involved in the fine control of sodium balance. It must be emphasized that aldosterone affects the renal tubular reabsorption of a small, albeit highly significant, fraction of the filtered sodium. This hormone stimulates reabsorption of sodium and enhances the secretion of potassium and hydrogen ion in the distal nephron. Aldosterone secretion has been shown to be responsive to a number of humoral factors including angiotensin II, ACTH, and the serum concentrations of potassium ions and sodium ions in the blood perfusing the adrenal glands.

Hydrocortisone. Although the patient with adrenal insufficiency has a dramatic renal wastage of sodium ion due to aldosterone deficiency, it is less well appreciated that a defect in excretion of dilute urine is also present which is not corrected by the administration of aldosterone or the replacement of sodium ion losses. The impairment of the diluting capacity is mainly due to an impairment of nephron function. In addition, some data suggest that inhibition of neurohypophyseal release of ADH may also be impaired. In the absence of hydrocortisone, the distal nephron becomes excessively permeable to water. In the presence of the normal medullary hypertonicity, water thus leaves the tubular lumen, even in the absence of ADH, at an excessive rate, thus concentrating the remaining solutes and impairing the renal diluting capacity. Any difficulty in inhibiting the secretion of ADH by normal osmotic and volume changes would also aggravate the renal diluting potential. The end result is the frequent development of water excess (hyponatremia) in patients with glucocorticoid deficiency. The administration of hydrocortisone to these patients will cause prompt dilution of the urine and excretion of the excess body water.

Parathyroid Hormone. Parathyroid hormone (parathormone) is one of several factors influencing the tubular excretion of phosphate. Parathormone secretion appears to be related to the concentration of ionic calcium perfusing the parathyroid glands. A reduction in the normal circulating concentration of ionic calcium will cause a release of the hormone, with its resultant effects on bone and kidney. The effect on bone is to increase the rate of bone resorption, resulting in an increase in circulating ionic calcium. The effect on the kidney is an increase in phosphate excretion and an increased reabsorption of calcium ion. The net result of all of these actions is to increase calcium ion and lower phosphate ion concentration in extracellular fluid.

Vasoactive Hormones. Angiotensin, epinephrine, and norepinephrine constrict renal vessels. When these substances are administered in moderate doses, a reduction in total renal blood flow as much as 50 percent, without significant change in GFR, is seen. The constancy of GFR is due to equal constriction of both afferent and efferent arterioles. When administered in higher doses, and especially when infused intravenously, these hormones cause a fall in both renal blood flow and filtration rate. Under these circumstances, afferent arteriolar constriction must be greater than efferent. In addition to their vascular action, these hormones also cause a striking decrease in renal excretion of sodium ion without changing the filtered load. It is probable that these direct effects on glomerulotubular balance are due to their action on peritubular blood flow. A possible interaction with the renin-angiotension-aldosterone system has also been suggested.

HORMONAL CONTROL OF BODY FLUID OSMOLALITY AND VOLUME

It is clear that the total volume and osmolality of the intracellular and extracellular compartments of body fluids are rigidly controlled, because only small fluctuations occur despite wide variations in dietary intake. Regulation of osmolality and volume in the extracellular compartment is accomplished by control of both intake and output. The *osmolality* of extracellular fluid depends primarily on water content. Gain of water induces prompt water diuresis; loss of water induces thirst and antidiuresis. The *volume* of extracellular fluid is regulated by control of the excretion of both sodium and water. Salt appetite and thirst are integral parts of both regulatory mechanisms, since deficits of sodium and water cannot be corrected merely by renal conservation. Since, in this country, the intake of sodium far exceeds the minimum need, regulation of salt intake normally plays very little part in maintaining the stability of extracellular fluid volume and composition.

Osmolal Regulation. The osmolality of extracellular fluid (280 ± 10 mOsm/L) is maintained primarily by regulation of the intake and excretion of water. Osmotic changes in the extracellular fluid are sensed by hypothalamic osmoreceptor cells, which regulate the release of ADH. The sensory mechanism is not entirely understood. In the past, these cells have been thought to respond as tiny osmometers, swelling when the extracellular fluid becomes hypotonic and shrinking when it becomes hypertonic. Shrinkage was presumed to stimulate neurogenic impulses which travel to the posterior pituitary, where ADH is stored and released. This may be over-simplified; recent data indicate that the important variant causing ADH release is the concentration of sodium in the cerebrospinal fluid (CSF) or extracellular space of the brain. This would explain the observation that direct instillation of non-electrolyte solutes such as sucrose and mannitol into the third ventricle of the brain does not stimulate ADH release although CSF osmolality is increased. In the light of this current concept, changes in ECF osmolality would regulate ADH release through the changes in CSF sodium concentration produced by shifts of water into or out of the brain and CSF.

The effect of ADH on the kidney is to increase the permeability of the distal portions of the nephron to water, thus increasing the reabsorption of water and rendering the urine hypertonic. This conservation of body water tends to bring the plasma back to its normal osmolality. This recovery is facilitated by thirst and an increased intake of water. Conversely, swelling of the osmoreceptors and/or a lowering of the concentration of CSF sodium inhibits the release of antidiuretic hormone. As circulating ADH is destroyed, the distal portions of the nephrons become less permeable to water and water is retained in the tubule, caus-

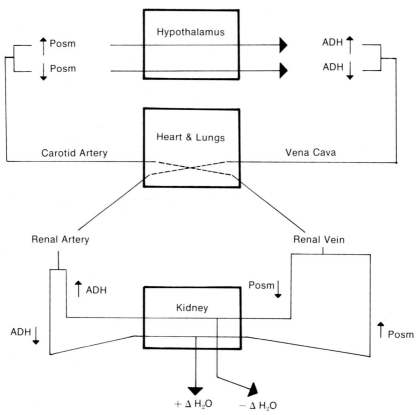

Figure 3–2. Control loop for osmoregulation. Explanation: Suppose that an existing balance between Na and water intake and excretion are disturbed such that plasma entering the carotid arteries becomes hyperosmotic (↑ Posm). The ADH level of the renal circulation increases (↑ ADH). Since Na^+ excretion is unchanged, urine osmolality increases while renal vein plasma osmolality decreases (↓ Posm). Mixture of renal venous blood with vascular pool (heart-lungs) decreases carotid artery and hypothalamic osmolality. This reduction in osmolality is sensed by hypothalamic osmoreceptors and the release of ADH from the pituitary decreases by an amount (↓ Posm) compared to the previous circulation cycle. A third cycle leads to further reduction in plasma osmolality and so on. Thus one may view the overall correction of an osmotic disturbance as taking place in a series of decreasing steps until the preferred osmolality is attained. Theoretically, the preferred osmolality is attained when renal artery ADH titer causes sufficient free water reabsorption to balance water losses and solute increases.

Table 3–1. Release of Antidiuretic Hormone

STIMULI	INHIBITORS
1. Osmotic	1. Osmotic
a. Contraction of intracellular volume secondary to hyper-osmolality of extracellular fluids (water loss)	a. Expansion of intracellular volume secondary to hypo-osmolality of the extracellular fluid (water ingestion)
2. Pressure-Volume	2. Pressure-Volume
a. Contraction of extracellular and/or plasma volume without alteration of osmolality	a. Expansion of extracellular and/or plasma volume without alteration of osmolality
b. Decreased intrathoracic blood volume (positive pressure breathing)	b. Increased intrathoracic blood volume (negative pressure breathing; CO_2 inhalation)
c. Upright position	c. Reclining position
3. Premonitory	3. Premonitory
a. Emotional stress	a. Emotional stress (occasionally)
b. Pain	b. Cold exposure
c. Drugs; anesthetics, opiates, barbiturates, nicotine, acetylcholine	c. Drug: acute alcohol ingestion

ing a dilute urine and a water diuresis. This tends to elevate plasma osmolality and bring it back toward normal (Figure 3–2).

Antidiuretic hormone release is enhanced or suppressed not only in response to changes in osmotic pressure of the body fluids but also in response to pressure-volume or premonitory stimuli (Table 3–1). Many observations suggest that moderate pressure-volume changes leave their prime effects on the low pressure side of the circulation. Receptors which sense these changes are mainly located in the left atrium, and signal the neurohypophyseal system through the vagus nerve.

The fact that a variety of stimuli affect release of ADH implies a central mechanism which receives afferent fibers from many sources, integrates the information transmitted over these pathways, and either inhibits or stimulates hormone secretion.

Volume Regulation. Preservation of a stable volume of extracellular fluid is a necessity for survival. Inasmuch as the bulk of osmotically active sodium within the body is confined to the ECF compartment, the extracellular volume is regulated directly by the renal control of sodium balance. Volume regulation involves receptors which sense errors in volume, neural and humoral mechanisms which apprise the kidney of those errors, and renal mechanisms by which the kidneys compensate for them. Volume receptors presumably are sensitive to ECF volume; to some fraction of that volume, such as plasma or interstitial fluid; to some derivative of volume, such as intravascular or interstitial pressure or distention; or to blood flow. Although some investigators believe that a single type of receptor responsive to a single stimulus activates mechanisms of volume control, it is probable that several types of receptors responsive to as many stimuli activate a number of effector mechanisms and provide defense in depth (see section on JGA, Chapter 2).

Renal mechanisms which compensate for errors in volume include those concerned with the excretion and conservation of sodium ion and water. Several mechanisms for the precise regulation of sodium ion excretion have been proposed: (1) GFR changes resulting in hemodynamic alterations in the sodium load presented to the renal tubules; (2) control of completeness of tubular reabsorption of sodium ion by variations in secretion of aldosterone by the adrenal cortex; and (3) control of completeness of tubular reabsorption by factors which are independent

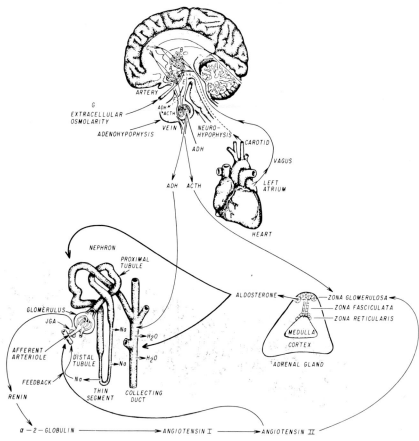

Figure 3-3. Integrative mechanisms for regulation of volume and osmolarity of the extracellular fluid. *A,* Osmoreceptors in supraoptic nucleus of hypothalamus; *B,* osmoreceptors in paraventricular nucleus of hypothalamus; *C,* stimuli to supraoptic and paraventricular nuclei from higher brain centers; *JGA,* juxtaglomerular apparatus, which secretes renin.

of changes in GFR or aldosterone secretion. These factors may be extrarenal hormonal influences or intrarenal physical changes.

Volume regulation is also mediated through the ADH system. Observations have shown that changes in ECF volume will have an effect on the stimulation or inhibition of ADH release. Two reservations must be stated about volume regulation through the ADH system. It is an emergency system which is called into play only in severe derangements. When it is active, osmolar regulation is sacrificed and extracellular fluid may become increasingly hypotonic.

A diagrammatic summary of some of the factors influencing osmolal and volume regulation of body fluids is seen in Figure 3–3.

DRUGS AND THE KIDNEY

Kinetics of Drug Excretion. Nearly all therapeutic drugs are eliminated from the body at a rate proportional to the amount of drug present in the body. A convenient way to express this rate of elimination is to measure the length of time needed for the plasma concentration of the drug to fall to one-half of its initial value. Although determination of the biologic half-life is simple, calculations based upon the value may be misleading because of various assumptions which do not always obtain.

For drugs excreted entirely by the kidney, the relationships between plasma half-life ($T_{1/2}$), its apparent volume of distribution (V), and clearance (C) of the drug from the body are illustrated in Figure 3–4.

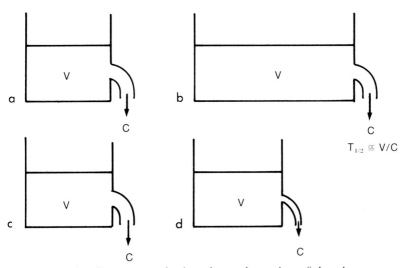

Figure 3–4. This diagram emphasizes the prolongation of the plasma concentration of a drug (an increase in $T_{1/2}$) which occurs with an increase in the volume of drug distribution (a vs b) or decrease in renal excretion (c vs d).

Table 3-2.   Interrelations Between Distribution Volume, Renal
Clearance, and Plasma Half-life.

DRUG	APPARENT VOLUME OF DISTRIBUTION, L	RENAL CLEARANCE, ML/MIN	PLASMA HALF-LIFE, MIN
A	3	120	18
B	12	120	70
C	42	120	245
D	42	600	48
E	42	30	980
F	1200	600	1440

The concept of apparent volume of distribution is primarily a mathematical concept used to relate the dose of a drug to the plasma concentration achieved by that dose. For certain drugs the mathematical distribution volume is equal to known body fluid compartment. For most drugs, however, the volume of distribution does not represent a discrete compartment but rather a heterogeneous distribution of the drug throughout the body. The importance of drug distribution and renal clearance is further demonstrated in Table 3-2, which underscores the influence of *both* parameters on the rate of elimination of a drug from the body.

Renal Excretion of Drugs.   The excretion of drugs and their active metabolites, an important factor in the determination of drug action, occurs via the kidneys, hepato-biliary system, intestine, and lungs. Renal excretion is quantitatively the most significant of these various routes. In the kidney, drugs are subjected to glomerular filtration, tubular reabsorption, tubular secretion, or a combination of secretion and reabsorption.

The excretion of a drug is highly dependent on GFR. Only that portion of a drug which is dissolved in the plasma water is freely filterable. Thus, the filtration of a compound is inversely proportional to its degree of protein binding. Most drugs are bound to plasma albumin so their filtration rate is less than the GFR.

Tubular secretion of drugs, an active transport process, takes place principally in the proximal tubule. Two different secretory mechanisms are involved: one for the elimination of organic acids such as PAH, chlorothiazide, penicillin, and probenecid, and the other for organic bases such as tetraethylammonium, histamine, and morphine. Concurrent administration of drugs which are excreted by a common secretory mechanism may affect the rates of secretion of one or both drugs, depending on their relative affinity for the transport mechanism. Experimentally, there are many examples of a weak acid slowing the secretion rate of another weak acid and weak bases slowing excretion of other weak bases. The use of probenecid to reduce penicillin secretion and thereby increase the plasma penicillin concentration is an example of this effect.

Table 3-3. Commonly Used Drugs Excreted Principally by the Kidneys.

Antibiotics	*Cardiovascular*
Aminosalicyclic Acid	Procainamide
Cephaloridine	Quinidine
Ethambutol	Methyldopa
Gentamicin	Digoxin
Isoniazid	Digitoxin
Kanamycin	Mercurials
Methenamine Mandelate	
Nitrofurantoin	*Miscellaneous*
Polymixins	Primidone
Spectinomycin	Trimethadione
Streptomycin	Azathioprine
Sulfasoxisole	Methotrexate
Vancomycin	Chlorpropamide
	Phenformin
Sedatives, Tranquilizers and Analgesics	Tolbutamide
Aspirin	Allopurinol
Phenobarbital	
Chlordiazepoxide	
Meprobamate	
Phenothiazines	
Phenylbutazone	

Because most drugs are weak acids or bases, they exist in plasma, water, and urine as only partially dissociated molecules. The ratio of un-ionized to ionized molecules is dependent on the pH of the solution and the dissociation constant (pK) of the acid or base concerned. As noted in Chapter 2 when discussing the NH_3 - NH_4^+ transport, un-ionized molecules which are lipid soluble diffuse more rapidly across the renal tubule than ionized particles which are water soluble. In clinical terms, this concept of non-ionic diffusion means that drugs which are weak acids will be excreted more rapidly in an alkaline urine (urine pH > drug pK) and weak bases excreted more rapidly in an acid urine.

Renal failure, by curtailing drug excretion, can increase the toxicity of many agents which are dependent on renal excretion as a major means for termination of action. A partial listing of drugs excreted predominantly by the kidney and which may require reduced doses in patients with renal failure is given in Table 3-3. The drugs most commonly implicated in toxic reaction in renal failure include digitalis and a number of antibiotics.

Renal Toxicity of Drugs. Toxic nephropathy is a general term used to describe any adverse functional or structural change in the kidney due to the effect of a chemical or biologic product which is inhaled, ingested, injected, or absorbed, or which yields toxic metabolites. Table 3-4 is one way of classifying nephrotoxic substances.

Table 3-5 represents a partial list of compounds which have been implicated in the past. Common clinical offenders include antibiotics, analgesics, organic solvents, and glycols.

Table 3-4. Classification of Nephrotoxins

1. Nephrotoxicity from a direct effect.
   a. Heavy metals
   b. Organic solvents
   c. Glycols
   d. Radiation
   e. Therapeutic drugs
   f. Insecticides

2. Nephrotoxicity from interaction of a toxin with other factors.
   a. Hypersensitivity reaction
   b. Hemolysis

3. Nephrotoxicity from abnormal concentrations of physiologic solutes.
   a. Hypercalcemia
   b. Hyperuricemia
   c. Hypokalemia

Drugs Affecting Renal Function (Diuretics). A positive sodium and water balance can only be produced by the kidney, although organs such as the gut and skin may play a role in producing sodium and water deficits. Renal handling of sodium is centered around two mechanisms: glomerular filtration and tubular reabsorption. Each of the clinically useful diuretics increases the excretion of sodium by diminishing reabsorption of this ion by the renal tubule rather than by increasing the amount of sodium filtered by the glomerulus. Normally the majority of tubular reabsorption takes place in the proximal convoluted segment of the nephron. This amounts to 70 percent of the sodium filtered. As less than 1 percent of the filtered sodium is excreted, the remaining 30 percent is reabsorbed in the loop of Henle, the distal convoluted tubule, and the collecting ducts. Micropuncture studies have shown that three-fourths of this sodium is reabsorbed in the loop of Henle.

Table 3-5. Nephrotoxic Compounds

Metals: mercury (organic and inorganic), bismuth, uranium, cadmium, lead, gold, arsine and arsenic, iron, silver, antimony, copper, and thallium.
Organic solvents: carbon tetrachloride, tetrachloroethylene, methyl cellosolve, methanol.
Glycols: ethylene glycol, ethylene glycol dinitrite, propylene glycol, ethylene dichloride, and diethylene glycol.
Physical agents: radiation, heat stroke, and electroshock.
Diagnostic agents: contrast agents in high concentration.
Therapeutic agents: Antibiotics: sulfonamides, penicillin, streptomycin, kanamycin, vancomycin, bacitracin, polymyxin, colistin, neomycin, tetracycline, cephloridine, gentamicin, and amphotericin. Analgesics: salicylates, para-aminosalicylate (PAS), phenacetin, phenylbutazone. Anti-convulsants: tridione, paradione.
Insecticides: biphenyl, chlorinated hydrocarbons.
Miscellaneous chemicals: carbon monoxide, snake venom, mushroom poison, spider venom, cresol, beryllium, hemolysins, aniline and other methemoglobin formers.

Diseases associated with edema produce pathologic stimuli which enhance sodium reabsorption in the proximal tubule and may also reduce glomerular filtration. The exact way in which this change in glomerulo-tubular balance is mediated, whether by hormonal or intrarenal mechanisms or both, is unknown. Whatever the mechanism, the development of edema probably requires the activation of both proximal and distal tubular reabsorption of sodium. Quantitatively, the more important of these mechanisms would be the one involving the proximal tubule. In the distal segment, sodium remaining in the tubule may be reabsorbed (without anions) if a reciprocal secretion of H^+ or K^+ occurs. This cation exchange is increased in response to (1) the rate at which sodium reaches this site, (2) the type of anions present, and (3) the degree of aldosteronism. An understanding of this exchange mechanism is important in understanding both the rationale for using various types of diuretics simultaneously and one of the major complications of diuretic therapy, potassium depletion and metabolic alkalosis.

The diuretics in general use can be divided conveniently into two groups. The first includes potent compounds, fully effective on their own, such as the organomercurials, thiazides, furosemide, and ethacrynic acid. The second group consists of agents not sufficiently potent to be diuretics of first choice but possessing qualities that may be valuable in supplementing or modifying the action of the major diuretics mentioned before. This latter group would include xanthines, osmotic agents, carbonic anhydrase inhibitors, aldosterone inhibitors, and triamterene.

Organomercurials. These agents reigned for 40 years after their introduction in 1920 as the only effective diuretics until the introduction of thiazides. They require parenteral administration, as no effective oral preparation is available. The site of action of mercurial diuretics is disputed, but the evidence indicates that their major effect in inhibiting sodium reabsorption lies beyond the proximal tubule. Knowledge of the mechanisms whereby these drugs impair active sodium transport is still fragmentary. The known affinity of inorganic mercury for sulphydryl groups suggests that organomercurials act by forming inactive complexes with sulphydryl-containing proteins and inactivating enzymes vital to electrolyte transport.

Mercurials result in the excretion of sodium and chloride in nearly equal amounts, which may result in metabolic alkalosis. The diuretic effectiveness of mercurials is lost in the presence of alkalosis and is enhanced by the intermittent administration of acidifying agents such as ammonium chloride or acetazolamide (Diamox). Under ideal conditions, these diuretics are quite potent and may cause excretion of 15 to 25 percent of the sodium filtered by the glomeruli. An additional property of clinical importance is their relative inhibition of potassium secretion. Despite marked interference with sodium reabsorption proximal to the site of sodium-potassium exchange, these agents do not result in depletion of potassium as rapidly as do the other potent diuretics.

The chief disadvantage of the mercurials is that they are only really satisfactory agents when given parenterally. Many patients, though appreciating the relief that they afforded, dreaded the frequent injections, and for them the advent of the orally effective thiazides, and more recently ethacrynic acid and furosemide, was an immense boon.

Nephrotoxic effects of organomercurials include both acute tubular necrosis and, rarely, the nephrotic syndrome. These usually follow prolonged high dosage in the presence of pre-existing kidney disease — an important contraindication to the use of mercurials.

Thiazides and Related Sulfonamides. The thiazide derivatives were the first potent orally effective diuretics. Although a large number of derivatives are available, certain general statements are applicable to each of these compounds including the non-thiazides, chlorthalidone (Hygroten) and quinethazone (Hydromox). When they are given in optimal dosage, the therapeutic action of saluresis and the undesirable side effects such as hyperuricemia and hyperglycemia are similar for all the derivatives; differences between the thiazides are limited largely to comparisons of potency on a weight basis, to the duration of effect, and to cost.

Originally, the action of chlorothiazide and its congeners was attributed to its carbonic anhydrase inhibitor activity; but this is relatively weak, and chlorothiazide produces a greater loss of chloride than bicarbonate in the urine. The diuretic effects are the result of direct interference with sodium reabsorption, and under optimal conditions may result in the excretion of approximately 5 percent of the sodium filtered. Thiazides appear to interfere with sodium reabsorption in the proximal tubule and loop of Henle. They appear to have a significant effect on the diluting segment of the nephron (probably the early distal tubule) and reduce renal diluting capacity. Sodium blockade in this site reduces the tubular diluting capacity. In contrast to organomercurials, the effect of thiazides on sodium excretion is not influenced by acid-base balance. Only oral preparations are commonly available. Thiazides have been very extensively used and have caused remarkably few serious toxic reactions.

The thiazides are effective agents in therapy of hypertension. Current evidence suggests that thiazides have a direct action on the blood vessels, quite apart from any hypotensive effect that may result from sodium depletion.

Furosemide and Ethacrynic Acid. These are relatively new orally effective, non-thiazide, non-mercurial diuretics which are extremely potent and appear to exert their major effect on sodium reabsorption on the proximal tubule in the loop of Henle. Both drugs are effective when given orally or parenterally, although ethacrynic acid cannot be given intramuscularly. The greater diuretic efficacy of these two compounds in blocking renal tubular sodium reabsorption is a most impressive phenomenon. Single doses of ethacrynic acid have caused the excretion of as much as 45 percent of filtered sodium load with loss of 18 pounds of body weight in the subsequent 24 hours. Like the thiazides, these drugs limit but do not abolish the ability to excrete dilute urine, and because of their action in the loop of Henle, they result in a marked impairment in the ability to concentrate urine. These agents will increase the excretion of potassium. Unlike the mercurials, these drugs do not lose their effectiveness in the presence of the electrolyte disturbances that they may produce. These include hyponatremia, hypopotassemia, and especially hypochloremic alkalosis. The major problems associated with these drugs are related to their pharmacological potency rather than to any true toxic effects. Rarely the acute loss of water and electrolytes may be so massive as to cause hypotension and collapse. Vascular thrombosis also can be precipitated. Presumably this is secondary to the disproportionate increase in blood viscosity that occurs when the hematocrit increases slightly. It must be realized that furosemide and ethacrynic acid may remain effective in the presence of gross electrolyte dislocations, hypoalbuminemia and a marked decrease in GFR. Nevertheless, a small proportion of patients still fail to respond even to these powerful drugs.

Because of their potency and rapidity of action, the intravenous use of these drugs can be especially rewarding in the treatment of emergency situations such as acute pulmonary edema and hypertensive crises, and oliguria. Diuresis as great as three liters can be produced in a four-hour period.

Xanthines. The three main naturally occurring members of this group are caffeine, theobromine, and theophylline. Aminophylline is a conjugate of theophylline and is the only xanthine currently employed as a diuretic. Ability to induce diuresis is but one minor facet of their widespread pharmacological properties, which include stimulation of the central nervous system and heart, dilatation of blood vessels and bronchioles. The diuretic effect can be ascribed to an enhancement of the cardiac output, local vasodilation of renal arterioles with an increase in renal blood flow, and an inhibition of proximal tubular sodium reabsorption. Under appropriate conditions, 1 to 2 percent of the filtered sodium may be excreted. By taking advantage of this agent's ability to increase glomerular filtration rate, it is often possible to restore responsiveness to other diuretics when this has lapsed because of a reduction in filtered electrolyte load.

Osmotic Diuretics. The action of these agents (urea, glucose, mannitol, etc.) has been classically ascribed to the presence of non-reabsorbable solute filtered at the glomerulus which increases the osmolality of tubular fluid and inhibits proximal reabsorption of sodium and water. The increased load of fluid and retained solute is then delivered at a high rate of flow to the distal parts of the nephron, where it overwhelms the resorptive capacity of these segments and is excreted in the urine. During an active diuresis, as much as 5 to 10 percent of the filtered sodium may be excreted. Because osmotic diuretics result in a greater water than sodium loss, prolonged use may result in water depletion with resultant hypernatremia and hyperosmolality. The most commonly used osmotic diuretic is mannitol. It is non-toxic, is not metabolized, and is excreted principally by glomerular filtration. Unfortunately, the benefit of the diuresis it may produce in congestive failure is outweighed by the frequent development of pulmonary edema. It is more valuable in various oliguric conditions, especially those occurring post-operatively.

Osmotic diuresis may be seen during the course of some clinical diseases such as uncontrolled diabetes mellitus. In this disease the hyperglycemia and increased filtered glucose exceed the renal tubular capacity for reabsorption, which causes an osmotic diuresis.

Carbonic Anhydrase Inhibitors. These compounds, the first orally effective diuretics, were discovered after it was found that sulfanilamide could cause diuresis. Unfortunately, they are of low potency and if continued daily, become virtually ineffective. Although not clinically important modern diuretics, these agents have historical importance for their contribution to our knowledge of ion transport in the kidney. Because they impair the hydration of carbon dioxide in tubular cells, the intracellular production of carbonic acid is reduced, resulting in a decrease in sodium and bicarbonate reabsorption in the proximal tubule, an alkaline urine, and an enhancement of potassium excretion in the distal tubule. Tubular secretion of ammonia is also impaired due to the alkalinity of tubular fluid. The end result is the production of metabolic acidosis. This acidosis and the prominent kaliuresis greatly limit its clinical usefulness. Certain extrarenal effects of these agents make them useful in treating some cases of glaucoma and epilepsy. Oral and intravenous preparations are available.

Aldosterone Antagonists and Triamterene. Both spironolactone (Aldactone), an aldosterone antagonist, and triamterene (Dyrenium) exert their major effect on inhibition of sodium reabsorption in the distal tubule. These agents also diminish the rate of potassium and hydrogen secretion. Since the distal tubular transport mechanism is stimulated by aldosterone, spironolactone will increase the excretion of sodium appreciably only when a significant amount of sodium reaches this distal site and reabsorption is being stimulated by aldosterone. Although triamterene does not appear to antagonize the action of aldosterone, it does block the exchange of sodium for potassium, and its effect on electrolyte excretion may be indistinguishable from that of spironolactone. The diuretic efficacy of triamterene also depends on the quantity of sodium being reabsorbed in the distal nephron in exchange for secreted potassium, but because of its lack of dependency upon a tubular effect of aldosterone, triamterene may be effective when spironolactone is not. These two agents are additive in their effects. Under optimal conditions 1 to 2 percent of the filtered sodium may be excreted. Only oral preparations are available.

Aldosterone antagonists are not useful as primary diuretics due to weakness of action, but they may be useful adjuvants to other diuretics by offsetting potassium depletion. The important potential untoward effect of these drugs is hyperpotassemia. Therefore, they should be given cautiously in patients with impaired renal function, and of course, potassium supplementation is contraindicated.

Complications

Disorders of Potassium. Potassium depletion is probably the most common complication of effective diuretic treatment. Since each of the potent diuretic agents interferes with sodium reabsorption proximal to the distal potassium secretory site, these agents result in increased delivery of sodium distally, and in the presence of varying concentrations of aldosterone result in increased secretion of potassium. One of the problems caused by potassium deficiency is the increased risk of digitalis intoxication during a diuretic-plus-glycoside regimen. A negative potassium balance may be prevented through dietary supplementation or by the simultaneous administration of spironolactone or triamterene to block potassium secretion. The latter alternative has the advantage of enhancing the excretion of sodium. The singular administration of spironolactone or triamterene results in the retention of potassium and may cause hyperkalemia.

Acid-Base Disturbances. The more potent diuretic agents increase the excretion of sodium and chloride in nearly equivalent amounts, which may result in metabolic alkalosis. This may not have clinical importance except for a reduction in the effectiveness of mercurial diuretics. This disturbance may be avoided by intermittent diuretic use or the administration of acidifying agents.

Hyperuricemia and Gout. Hyperuricemia due to a reduced urate clearance is a common complication of thiazide, furosemide, and ethacrynic acid treatment. This secondary hyperuricemia rarely results in symptomatic gout in the non-gouty patient and is responsive to uricosuric agents.

Hyperglycemia and Diabetes Mellitus. The decreased glucose tolerance produced by thiazides appears to be caused by a reduction in both the release of insulin and the utilization of glucose in the peripheral tissues. This complication may worsen the control of the diabetic patient but is readily overcome by appropriate adjustment of the anti-diabetic treatment. There is no evidence that the hyperglycemic effect of thiazides has produced frank diabetes in persons not predisposed to the disorder.

Hyponatremia. Even in the presence of residual edema or ascites, the forced renal excretion of sodium not infrequently results in a syndrome indistinguishable in some aspects from volume depletion.

Under these circumstances, renal function may deteriorate, urine volume may become scanty, and ingested water will be retained, resulting in progressive hyponatremia. Although this same complex of abnormalities occur spontaneously in far advanced stages of edema, when these disorders appear in the course of diuretic treatment they should be regarded as unequivocal indications to discontinue diuresis despite the presence of residual edema.

General Considerations. Diuretics can only relieve a symptom. They do not remove the underlying cause, though the dispersal of edema may in turn have secondary beneficial effects such as better arterial oxygenation and improvement of the circulation. Nevertheless, it is possible to pay too high a price in the attempt to gain complete symptomatic relief. Excessive diuretic therapy may, in spite of the persistence of some edema, lead to a rising blood urea, serious electrolyte disturbances, hepatic coma, and the hyponatremic state.

After the initial three to four consecutive days of therapy, it is often preferable to give diuretics, particularly the more powerful ones, in an

Table 3-6. Diuretics Currently Useful

TYPE	NON-PROPRIETARY	TRADE NAME
Mercurials	mercaptomerin	Thiomerin
	meralluride	Mercuhydrin
	mercurophylline	Mercuzanthin
	mersalyl	Salyrgan
	merethoxylline	Dicurin
	chlormerodrin	Neohydrin
Carbonic Anhydrase Inhibitors	acetazolamide	Diamox
	ethoxzolamide	Cardrase
	methazolamide	Neptazane
Thiazides	chlorothiazide	Diuril
	hydrochlorothiazide	Esidrix, Hydrodiuril, Oretic
	bendroflumethiazide	Benuron, Naturetin
	benzthiazide	Aquatag, Exna
	cyclothiazide	Anhydron
	hydroflumenthiazide	Saluron
	methylclothiazide	Enduron
	polythiazide	Renese
	trichlormethiazide	Metahydrin, Naqua
	flumethiazide	Ademol
Thiazide-Related Sulfonamides	chlorthalidone	Hygroton
	quinethazone	Hydromox
Potassium-Sparing Agents	spironolactone	Aldactone
	triamterene	Dyrenium
Others	ethacrynic acid	Edecrin
	furosemide	Lasix

intermittent rather than daily regimen. This allows time for the natural correction of electrolyte imbalances and other side effects.

Failure to achieve a response to potent diuretics may be due to diminished glomerular filtration, and it is important to look at extrarenal factors that may require attention, such as the treatment of pulmonary infection, the adequacy of bed rest, the correction of potassium depletion, and the proper use of digitalis.

Table 3–6 lists a number of the diuretics presently in use and their trade names.

DRUGS AFFECTING BLADDER FUNCTION

The two most important drugs that affect the bladder are those that stimulate the bladder detrusor muscle (cholinergics, parasympathomimetics) and those which inhibit the bladder detrusor muscle (anticholinergics, parasympatholytics).

The most effective and widely used cholinergic drugs are the stable choline esters (methacholine chloride, beta-methylcholine chloride). These drugs have the same action as the labile acetylcholine, that is, on the smooth muscle fibers of the bladder itself. These drugs are used to increase the muscle tone and to increase the force of contraction at micturition. Their effectiveness is difficult to predict on any given patient, but they have been used with success in patients with large bladder capacities who do not void completely or are prone to infection due to residual urine and the long time between voidings; patients with sensory deficits as in diabetes and syphilis; patients with brain or spinal cord lesions with resultant paresis or hemiparesis; and patients with large bladders after distention due to bladder neck obstruction. The most effective drug seems to be beta-methylcholine chloride. It is given orally, with the dosage being varied depending on clinical results and the occurrence of side effects (sweating, abdominal cramps, and anxiety). The drug can be given parenterally; although this route produces a rapid onset, there is a high percentage of side effects.

The parasympatholytic drugs are used to relax or decrease the tone of the bladder muscle. The increased tone may be due to prolonged partial obstruction of the bladder with resultant detrusor hypertrophy and irritability (see Chapter 5); spinal cord or brain lesions resulting in a spastic type neurogenic bladder contraction; acute or chronic irritation seen in bladder calculi, indwelling catheters, and post-instrumentation reaction; cystitis; genitourinary tuberculosis; or post-irradiation reaction of the bladder. The most common drug of this type is atropine. It blocks the post-ganglionic actions of acetylcholine. Although atropine is a component of many "bladder sedatives," its associated side effects make it less desirable than the more frequently used quaternary amines, meth-antheline bromide and propantheline bromide.

In treating patients with partial or compensated bladder obstruc-tion, it must be borne in mind that many anti-Parkinsonian drugs, antihistamines, and tranquilizers have a relaxing effect on the bladder. Thus, a history of the type of medication taken is of prime importance in the patient with suspected bladder neck obstruction. Changing the drug or eliminating it may relieve the symptoms and signs of what was thought to be a pure anatomic obstruction.

Chapter 4

DIAGNOSIS AND TREATMENT OF FLUID AND ELECTROLYTE IMBALANCES

Pure water is certainly of all others the most salutary beverage.

TOBIAS SMOLLET (1721–1771)

Salt is white and pure,—there is something holy in salt.

NATHANIEL HAWTHORNE (1804–1864)

Potassium is of the soil and not the sea; it is of the cell but not the sap.

WALLACE O. FENN (1893–   )

In all things you shall find everywhere the Acid and the Alcaly.

OTTO TACHENIUS (–1670)

Disturbances of fluid and electrolyte balance tend to occur whenever a patient becomes seriously ill from almost any cause. Obviously, if large amounts of body fluid are lost through vomiting and diarrhea, the disturbance can be acute, severe, and even fatal. Whenever the heart, kidneys or lungs are diseased and malfunctioning, fluid imbalance is particularly prone to develop since these are the prime movers and regulators of the internal environment.

Although seldom listed as a cause of death, fluid-electrolyte imbalance may contribute greatly to morbidity in the seriously ill patient and, if neglected, cause an unfavorable outcome. Fluid, electrolyte, and nutritional imbalances are like old age—they seldom cause trouble themselves, but often predispose to trouble. The sicker the patient, the

89

poorer his cardiac, respiratory, or renal reserve, the more important the maintenance of fluid-electrolyte balance becomes in preventing morbidity and mortality.

PHYSIOLOGICAL CONTROL OF WATER AND SODIUM

Water Balance—Regulation of Body Osmolality.   On a daily basis, a typical individual will imbibe 2500 ml of water and lose an equal amount, mostly as urine, but also a significant fraction through sweating and breathing (sensible and insensible losses) and a smaller fraction as stool moisture (Figure 4–1).

The regulation of body water is essentially the regulation of body osmolality. Osmolality is defined as the number of active solutes per unit of water. The electrolytes of the body contribute the largest number of solutes, with the most important being sodium and chloride in ECF and potassium and phosphate in ICF. Because of the free movement of water, intracellular and extracellular osmolalities are equal and the term "body osmolality" is permissible.

Body osmolality could be regulated by alteration of either water or solute content. Normally, osmolality is controlled quite precisely (±3 mOsm/kg) by regulation of water balance, thirst altering intake and ADH adjusting renal losses (Chapter 3).

Measurements of osmolality can be made by several methods, but the determination of the freezing point depression (Chapter 1) with an osmometer is the most accurate. Body osmolality is determined through measurement of the plasma osmolality (Posm) directly with an osmometer or indirectly by the *plasma sodium concentration*. Plasma sodium

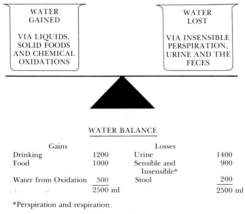

WATER BALANCE

	Gains		Losses	
Drinking	1200	Urine	1400
Food	1000	Sensible and Insensible*	900
Water from Oxidation	300	Stool	200
	2500 ml		2500 ml

*Perspiration and respiration

Figure 4–1.

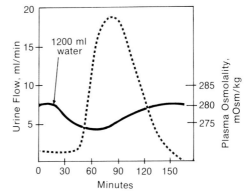

Figure 4-2. Water load.

concentration measures approximately one-half of the total osmolality (the other one-half being the total associated anions) because over 90 percent of the total cations in this fluid compartment are sodium. The total osmolality consists mostly of the ionized solutes, since non-ionized substances such as glucose and urea contribute few solutes in relation to the total number in healthy subjects. However, certain diseases such as diabetes mellitus (hyperglycemia) and uremia (elevation of plasma urea) may alter this simple relationship. Since most plasma cations and anions are monovalent, contributing one solute for each ion, measurement of one-half of the ions is a reasonably accurate reflection of plasma osmolality. Therefore, *when plasma glucose and urea concentrations are normal,* the following relationship pertains:

$$\text{Posm} = [\text{Na}^+]_p \times 2$$
$$\text{(mOsm/kg)} \quad \text{(mEq/L)}$$

Hyposmolality indicates an excess of water relative to solute, and hyperosmolality indicates a decrease in water relative to solute. An individual whose water intake exceeds water excretion develops water excess. Correspondingly, an individual who loses more water than imbibed becomes water depleted.

During water depletion, urine flow rate will decrease to 0.3 to 0.5 ml/min and urine concentration will exceed 1000 mOsm/kg. The renal response to an increase in *free water** is to increase water excretion. For example, an individual in water balance may be producing 1 ml/min of urine with an osmolality of 600 mOsm/kg. Upon drinking one liter of water, Posm falls, ADH release is inhibited, and urine production may increase to 10 to 15 ml/min with a fall in urine osmolality to 50 to 100

---

*A 300 mOsm/kg solution of sodium chloride (150 mEq/L) has a balance of water and solute which is isosmotic to plasma. A hyposmotic solution contains an excess of water ("free water") relative to solute. For example, 2 liters of a 150 mOsm/kg solution of sodium chloride (75 mEq/L) contains 1 liter of free water. Although a 5% glucose solution is also isotonic, it is entirely "free water" because the glucose is rapidly metabolized in the body.

mOsm/kg. Within a couple of hours, the liter of water will have been excreted and the body water content and osmolality returned to normal (Figure 4–2).

Sodium Balance – Regulation of Extracellular Volume. The principal cation of the ECF is sodium, and its concentration in the ECF determines the effective osmotic pressure of the interstitial fluid and, hence, cellular hydration. There are about 80 mEq/kg in a normal adult or about 5600 mEq of sodium in a 70 kg individual. About 45 percent of this body sodium is in the ECF. A large amount of sodium is contained in bone, but only one-half of this is freely exchangeable with sodium in the ECF (Figure 4–3).

The average individual consumes about 50 to 200 mEq of sodium daily. With a constant intake of sodium, an equal amount is excreted each day, mostly in the urine, with a variable amount in sweat and a small fraction in the stool. If sodium intake exceeds excretion, a positive balance develops. This might be a short-term imbalance resulting from a salty meal or a chronic imbalance resulting from renal dysfunction. The effect on body fluids is the same in either case. The excess sodium (plus anion) which is confined to the ECF raises its osmolality; water rapidly diffuses from the ICF until osmotic equilibrium is restored. The net effect is to expand the ECF at the expense of cellular water and raise body osmolality. The rise in osmolality stimulates receptors in the hypothalamus, leading to a stimulation of thirst and a release of ADH. Body osmolality and cellular water are, thus, restored but at the expense of a further increase in ECF. This effect could have been achieved in one

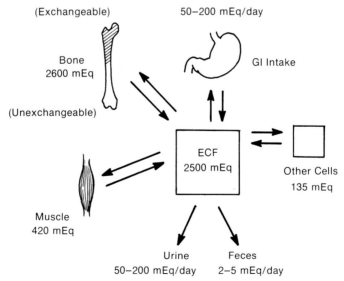

Figure 4–3. Sodium balance in a 70 kg subject.

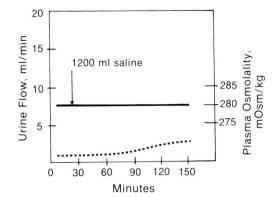

Figure 4–4. Isotonic saline load.

step by drinking isotonic saline containing an amount of sodium equal either to that in the salty meal or to that retained due to renal dysfunction.

The body is keenly aware of its ECF (Chapter 3) and the normal person would soon restore his ECF to normal by excreting the excess sodium and a commensurate amount of water. However, the excretion of a sodium load is notably slower than the excretion of a water load (Figure 4–4). Failure of the urinary system to excrete the daily sodium load results in excessive ECF expansion. A failure of sodium excretion may occur for any of a variety of reasons, but a decreased plasma volume, decreased cardiac output, or inadequate extracellular volume are the most frequent causes. On the other hand, when sodium losses exceed intake, negative sodium balance occurs. This might result from either urinary or gastrointestinal losses. The sodium deficit shrinks the volume of ECF and the kidney responds by reducing sodium (and water) excretion. It is well to point out that a sodium restricted diet in the normal subject is well tolerated as under these circumstances all sodium may be removed by the tubules from the glomerular filtrate.

Plasma Volume vs. ECF.   It is most important to realize that ECF and plasma volume can vary in opposite directions. Since plasma volume is part of the ECF, changes in the extracellular space always have an effect on plasma volume. However, it should be recalled (Chapter 1) that the fraction of ECF formed by plasma depends on plasma protein concentration. Thus, an abnormal concentration of plasma proteins produces a proportional disturbance in the plasma volume. It is possible in hypoproteinemia, for example, for the plasma volume to decrease when the ECF is increasing. The particular relationship between plasma volume and ECF which exists will depend on the pathological factors affecting body sodium, plasma proteins, and other factors affecting fluid exchange across capillaries.

DISTURBANCES OF SODIUM AND WATER BALANCE

The determination of sodium and water need in the past has been a difficult aspect of the care of the sick patient. The problem will be discussed here on the physiological hypothesis that sodium disorders are extracellular volume disorders and water disorders are osmolality disorders.

Terminology. Because it is often used to mean some combination of disorders of sodium and water balance, the term "dehydration" often causes confusion. The terms *saline excess* and *saline depletion* avoid confusion by emphasizing the importance of the volume changes in sodium disturbances. Some physicians may find the term "saline" unsatisfactory. Any such term is satisfactory which conveys the idea that sodium disorders are volume disorders involving deficits or excesses of isotonic sodium solutions. The corrective therapy for these disorders is implied by the diagnostic terms *saline excess* and *saline depletion.*

Disturbances of water balance are defined as disturbances of osmolality. Low plasma osmolality, as indicated by decreased plasma sodium concentration (hyponatremia), is termed *water excess;* both extracellular and intracellular water are increased in relation to solute, the cells being overhydrated. Increased plasma osmolality associated with an elevated plasma sodium concentration (hypernatremia) is termed *water depletion.* The extracellular compartment and the cells are underhydrated. It must clearly be understood that disorders of water balance depend only on the relative amounts of water and solute present and not on the absolute amount of total body water. Thus, a patient with edema (saline excess) may have an increase in total body water; but since the retained sodium and water are isotonic and are located in the extracellular space, there is no change in intracellular water and, therefore, no disorder of water balance.

Disturbances of Sodium Balance

Using the extracellular volume as the guide to sodium requirements simplifies the therapeutic approach but emphasizes the difficulties inherent in the estimation of that volume. Fortunately, modest variations in extracellular volume are not harmful to most patients. Combined use of history, physical examination, hematocrit, plasma protein, and urine sodium or chloride permits detection of significant changes in extracellular volume (Figure 4–5).

Saline Depletion. Any patient with a decrease in extracellular volume is, by definition, saline depleted. (The slight decrease in extracellular volume that occurs with severe water depletion is not considered saline depletion.) The principal routes for loss of sodium from the

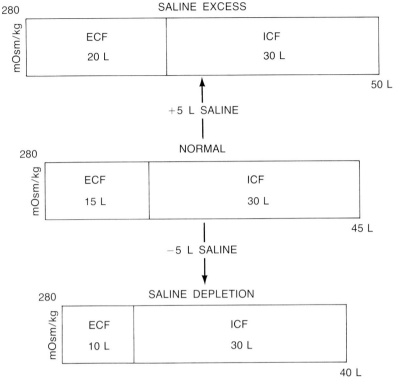

Figure 4–5.   Distribution of saline excess and depletion.

body can best be grouped into renal and extrarenal causes, as in Table 4–1.

The single most important criterion in the diagnosis of saline depletion is a HISTORY OF LOSS OF SODIUM-CONTAINING FLUID.

Table 4–1.   Causes of sodium depletion.

I. Renal losses
   A. No intrinsic renal disease
      1. Osmotic diuresis (glycosuria, mannitol infusion, etc.)
      2. Diuretic drugs (thiazides, ethacrynic acid, furosemide, mercurials)
      3. (Primary) adrenal insufficiency
      4. (Primary) inappropriate secretion of ADH
   B. Intrinsic renal disease
      1. Chronic renal disease (particularly medullary cystic disease and interstitial nephritis)
      2. Diuretic phase of "acute tubular injury"
      3. Post-obstructive uropathy
II. Extrarenal losses
   A. Gastrointestinal: vomiting, diarrhea, bowel drainage or fistula
   B. Skin: sweating, burns
   C. Iatrogenic: paracentesis, thoracentesis

The history has both a positive and negative value in diagnosis. On the positive side, any patient who gives a history of vomiting, diarrhea, or excessive sweating or has renal salt-wasting should be suspect. On the negative side, if a diagnosis of saline depletion has been made, absence of a history of loss of sodium-containing fluid makes the diagnosis extremely tenuous. These principles are based on the fact that when sodium intake ceases, the normal kidney can conserve sodium so well that clinically detectable saline depletion does not develop. Hence, unless the patient actually loses sodium-containing fluids, he will not become saline depleted.

The *symptoms and signs* of saline depletion are primarily those of an *inadequate blood volume* resulting from ECF losses. Initial symptoms of anorexia, nausea, weakness, and giddiness may be followed by orthostatic syncope, fainting, and finally, circulatory collapse. It is important to emphasize that even though these findings suggest the presence of an inadequate blood volume, they do not prove the existence of saline depletion. A number of conditions, including blood loss, septic shock, and myocardial infarction, must first be excluded. In the case of the differential between saline depletion and blood or plasma depletion, measurement of the plasma protein concentration is helpful. If the hypovolemia is due to pure saline depletion, the plasma protein concentration will be elevated; if it is not, the plasma protein deficiency is, at least in part, responsible for the hypovolemia.

Of the various signs of an inadequate blood volume, *postural changes in blood pressure* are among the most sensitive. When trying to elicit this diagnostic sign, it is important to measure the blood pressure first with the patient supine and then after sitting on the edge of the bed or standing. Merely sitting up in bed is insufficient postural change to elicit the sign. Normally, when a patient changes from the lying to the sitting or standing position, his systolic pressure changes very little and his diastolic pressure rises about 5 to 10 mm Hg. In the presence of an inadequate blood volume, the systolic and diastolic pressures fall 10 mm Hg or more. A slight fall in systolic pressure alone does not indicate an inadequate blood volume.

Significant postural hypotension will occur in the presence of severe peripheral autonomic nervous system disease and in some cardiac patients with relatively fixed cardiac output. However, the postural drop that often is found in any patient who has been bedridden for a long time usually indicates an inadequate blood volume associated with a decrease in ECF. Severe postural hypotension is a common cause of fainting with injuries, cerebrovascular accidents, or coronary occlusion under these circumstances, especially among older people.

Learning to "read" *neck veins* can prove useful in the assessment of blood volume disorders. When a patient lies absolutely flat on his back in bed, his neck veins should be full nearly to the angle of the jaw. If the bed must be raised to an angle before a level can be seen, then the pressure is increased and circulatory overload should be suspected. The finding of decreased filling or *flat neck veins* which fill only when compressed at the clavicles strongly suggests an inadequate blood volume.

In many patients, especially those with a thick neck, neck veins either are absent or are difficult to find. Furthermore, the blood volume may be inadequate in the presence of normally full neck veins. Hence, in some patients, direct measurement of *central venous pressure* (CVP) is necessary and warranted provided the well-known risks associated with the use of indwelling catheters are recognized and minimized by proper technique.

Contrary to earlier convictions and despite common opinion, direct measurement of CVP is not a good sign of an inadequate blood volume because the range of normality is so wide. Furthermore, measurements of CVP do not correlate well with fullness of neck veins due to variation in a number of factors including venous tone. The value of CVP lies in noting pressure changes as volume replacement proceeds. In a patient with signs of an inadequate blood volume, *serial measurement* of CVP can help guide therapy, especially in complex problems involving combinations of shock, myocardial failure, pulmonary disease, and sepsis. The general principles pertaining to the interpretation of CVP are as follows:

1. A low CVP cannot be used as conclusive evidence of a low blood volume or circulatory insufficiency (shock).
2. In a patient with circulatory insufficiency:
    a. A low normal CVP indicates that the response to volume expansion should be immediately beneficial.
    b. A high CVP does not of itself contraindicate volume expansion. However, the venous pressure should remain constant or fall as the blood volume increases.
    c. If the initial CVP is elevated and rises further with volume expansion, such therapy is harming the patient and should be discontinued.
3. Any sustained rise above normal in CVP during volume replacement indicates that expansion may be excessive.

If the above principles are followed, the production of pulmonary congestion by volume expansion will be avoided, since rises in CVP are usually seen before increases in left ventricular end diastolic pressure (a sign of left ventricular failure).

As can be judged from the above discussion, CVP is not easy to interpret without considerable experience. Another indication of the adequacy of blood volume is the *hourly urine volume*. However, its value is limited in that oliguria may be caused by a wide variety of problems. The circumstances in which urine volume is most helpful are the following:

1. If during volume replacement there is an increase in hourly urine volume from oliguirc levels of 0 to 10 ml/hr up to 50 ml/hr

or more, this strongly indicates that an adequate blood volume
has been restored.

2. In patients who are losing blood volume rapidly (GI bleeding
or severe burns), a drop in the hourly urine volume usually
indicates that volume replacement is not keeping abreast of
continuing losses.

To recapitulate, if the patient has saline depletion and does not have
severe sepsis or cardiac disease, the signs of an inadequate blood volume
(postural hypotension and collapsed neck veins) are sensitive indices of
saline depletion. The same can be said for simple blood and plasma
depletion. It is only in patients critically ill with combinations of septic
shock, myocardial failure, and pulmonary dysfunction that these findings become difficult to detect and interpret. In such instances monitor-
ing the CVP and hourly urine volume is indicated.

The so-called classic physical signs of saline depletion, *decreased
skin turgor, shrunken tongue*, and *collapse of the anterior chamber of the eye*, are
actually of very little clinical value. It is difficult to be sure that these signs
are actually present, since wasting disease can closely mimic changes in
skin turgor. And, in order for these signs to be readily detectable, saline
depletion must be so severe that the patient is nearly in frank shock.

An elevated hematocrit and protein concentration are consistent
with the diagnosis of saline depletion, since plasma volume shares in the
loss of extracellular volume. If severe, renal function may be impaired,
especially in infants.

Urinary sodium or chloride excretion is an easily obtained and valuable
guide to the sodium needs of the patient. When a normal subject is
deprived of sodium, a fall in urine sodium and chloride occurs within
three days and is an early indication of extracellular volume contraction.
Hence, in the presence of normal renal function and the absence of
diuretic treatment, a urinary sodium concentration of 10 mEq/L or
greater or a chloride concentration greater than 50 mEq/L suggests that
the patient either does not have saline depletion, has been volume
depleted for less than three days, or does not conserve sodium normally.
The only exceptions to these observations are encountered when chloride
concentration is measured alone. First, there are occasional patients with
severe acidosis and mild saline depletion who will be excreting moderate
amounts of chloride (not sodium) in association with ammonium ions. In
the same general category are patients losing sodium-containing gastrointestinal fluid which is replaced largely as ammonium and potassium
chloride. A direct measurement of urinary sodium will avoid these exceptions.

It is important to remember that most patients with chronic renal
failure are unable to conserve sodium normally. When renal insufficiency is severe (plasma creatinine > 5 mg/100 ml), sodium wastage
may be a major problem, even leading to severe saline depletion if
dietary intake is inadequate.

A low urine sodium or chloride is not diagnostic of sodium depletion because it may result from nothing more than a low salt intake or an enlarging extracellular volume in diseases such as heart or liver failure. When considered in relation to intake, a low urine sodium or chloride often is the earliest manifestation of such an abnormal physiologic process.

Treatment of saline depletion consists of giving more isotonic sodium solution than required for maintenance therapy. The more certain the evidence that saline depletion is present, the more vigorous replacement therapy should be. While it is quite true that acute pulmonary edema may result from too rapid administration of saline, it is equally true that unnecessary prolongation of hypovolemia by too slow replacement of a saline deficit can have disastrous consequences, especially if the patient is stressed by surgery or hemorrhage. In the presence of saline depletion, intravenous administration of saline can proceed as rapidly as a liter per hour or in severe cases even faster, provided that the physician monitors the CVP frequently. As soon as the signs of severe hypovolemia begin to disappear, the rate of saline replacement is slowed and gradually allowed to drop to basic allowance levels.

It really is not necessary to quantitate the degree of saline depletion except very roughly. Severe depletion represents a 40 to 50 percent decrease in the ECF, while 25 to 30 percent depletion is considered moderate. If one assumes that the ECF normally is 20 percent of the body weight, actual rough quantitation is possible and provides a guide to the magnitude of the correction required.

For infants the extracellular volume is estimated as 20 to 25 percent of the normal body weight, and deficits of one-fourth to one-half commonly occur. Therefore, correction allowances of 20 to 50 ml of isotonic sodium repair solutions* per kg of body weight are made during the first period. Smaller amounts are used in subsequent periods to avoid the risk of overexpansion of extracellular volume during therapy as a result of inexact estimation of the volume deficit.

Saline Excess.   This disorder is, by definition, an increase above normal in the volume of the sodium space of the body, and, if great enough, is manifest as edema. It usually occurs in patients with *cardiac, hepatic,* and *renal disease* or with *severe protein depletion* from any cause. Regrettably, it also occurs on an iatrogenic basis. The physical findings are weight gain and, later, edema. Peripheral edema usually produces few symptoms, with patients complaining of tight shoes or ankle swelling. The increase in extracellular volume which must occur before edema is apparent depends mainly on tissue elasticity and posture. An elderly patient in a chair can have ankle edema with very little increase,

---

*In infants the renal ability to excrete acid is limited and catabolic acid load is relatively high. Thus, it is usually necessary to give a combination sodium bicarbonate and chloride as determined by the degree of acidosis.

while a supine patient can have an increase in volume of 4 to 8 liters without detectable peripheral edema. The periorbital edema in children found in the morning commonly disappears shortly after arising. Pulmonary edema is life threatening but usually develops after significant peripheral edema has collected. In some diseases such as heart failure and shock it may appear relatively early.

The hematocrit is often normal because saline excess develops rather slowly and compensatory factors maintain the hematocrit. The urine sodium or chloride is usually low, because the same factors which cause edema also cause renal retention of sodium and chloride. Were it not for renal retention of sodium, the disorder would quickly be corrected. As in saline depletion, the serum sodium concentration is normal unless a combined disorder exists.

In addition to treatment of the underlying cause, whether it be heart failure, hypoproteinemia, or some other problem, sodium restriction and diuretics often are indicated.

Body Weight as a Guide to Saline Need.   Changes in body weight over a short period of time measure changes in total body water. Hence, in order to use body weight as a guide to saline need, a way of calculating changes in ECF from the observed change in body weight must be formulated. The following equation indicates the factors causing changes in body weight.

$$\Delta Wt = \Delta ECF + \Delta ICF + \Delta Fat \text{ and Protein Mass}$$

Since ΔECF is the desired measurement, a method of estimating ΔICF and Δ Fat and Protein Mass is needed.

To estimate ΔICF, two assumptions are necessary. First, the ICF can be estimated as about 40 percent of the body weight. Second, changes in the ICF are proportional to changes in plasma osmolality (plasma sodium concentration).

$$\Delta ICF = (ICF)(\Delta[Na^+]_p) = (0.4 \times Body\ wt.) \left(\frac{Initial - Final\ [Na^+]_p}{Initial\ [Na^+]_p} \right)$$

Example:

Wt.: Initial 70 kg, Final 80 kg
Plasma sodium concentration: Initial 140 mEq/L, Final 126 mEq/L

$$\Delta Wt = \Delta ECF + \Delta ICF$$

$$+10 = \Delta ECF + \left(\frac{140 - 126}{140} \times 0.4 \times 70 \right)$$

$$+10 = \Delta ECF + 2.8$$
$$\Delta ECF = +7.2 \text{ liters}$$

An estimation of a change in the body fat and protein mass is made by assuming a loss of body weight of 0.3 kg/day for the catabolism that typically occurs when patients are ill and receiving only parenteral nutrition. In very catabolic individuals this loss may be as great as 0.6 kg/day.

Example:

	Weight	*Plasma Sodium*
Feb. 1	70 kg	130 mEq/L
Feb. 5	70 kg	130 mEq/L

$$\Delta Wt = \Delta ECF + \Delta ICF + \Delta \text{Fat and Protein Mass}$$

$$0 = \Delta ECF + 0 + (-0.3 \text{ kg/day} \times 4)$$

$$\Delta ECF = +1.2 \text{ liters}$$

The "Third Space" Problem.   Local factors may cause a sequestration of extracellular fluid as happens with thrombophlebitis, in a burned area, or in the lumen of an obstructed intestine. Such an accumulation of extracellular fluid has been termed a "third space," and represents loss of isotonic sodium-containing fluid from the normal extracellular space. The normal physiologic response decreases renal sodium excretion and returns the functional extracellular volume to normal. It is important that the weight gain and sodium and water retention which accompany a third space not be mistaken for an increase in extracellular volume and treated as such with sodium restriction or diuretics, because the result will be a reduction in the functional extracellular volume and plasma hypovolemia with little decrease in the third space.

Disturbances of Water Balance

The diagnosis and treatment of disturbances of water balance are relatively simple. Water administration is adjusted to maintain the plasma osmolality near normal (280 ± 10 mOsm/kg). This would be equivalent to a plasma sodium concentration between 135 and 145 mEq/L. Thus, plasma osmolality or sodium concentration (Figure 4–6) becomes the only necessary guide to water need, and its accurate measurement becomes very important.

Although freezing point depression could be used to measure plasma osmolality, it is more convenient to use the plasma sodium concentration as an index of body osmolality. Numerically, the body osmolality is almost exactly twice the measured plasma sodium level, but the calculation is seldom made and the serum sodium level itself is used as the guide to water dosage.

Since great reliance is placed on the plasma sodium concentration in determining the patient's need for water, it is of value to understand the

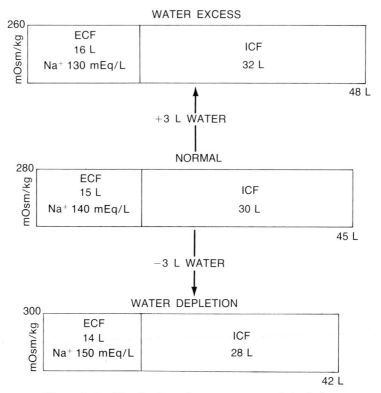

Figure 4–6. Distribution of water excess and depletion.

interrelationship between plasma sodium, chloride, and bicarbonate. Such an understanding provides an internal check on the validity of the laboratory measurements. This relationship is defined by the following equation:

$$[Na^+] = [Cl^-]_p + [HCO_3^-] + 10$$
$$140 = (105 + 25 + 10)$$

The factor 10, as shown in Figure 4–7, is the difference between the concentration of plasma sodium and that of the monovalent anions which are customarily measured. This cation-anion difference is called the *anion gap,* and it averages about 10 mEq/L. It mainly represents unmeasured anions derived from organic and inorganic acid metabolism. In addition to providing an internal check on the validity of the measured electrolytes, it is also apparent that certain types of metabolic acidosis may be predicted by the presence of an elevated anion gap. As shown in Figure 4–7, certain disease states cause accumulation of unmeasured anions, and a knowledge of this fact permits use of the anion

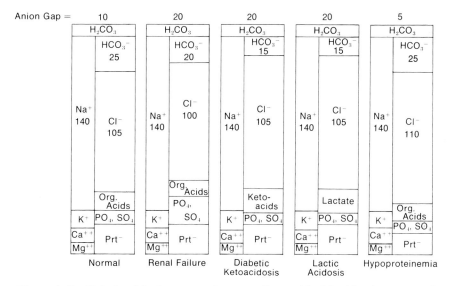

Figure 4-7. Relationship between plasma sodium, chloride, bicarbonate, and anion gap = sodium − (chloride + bicarbonate) in various diseases.

gap in recognizing and diagnosing possible causes for metabolic acidosis. With the exception of ketoacidosis and lactic acidosis, clinical states which are rapidly treated when recognized, the anion gap usually remains reasonably constant and can be used to check the validity of serial measurements of plasma electrolytes. Because the anion gap is influenced by the negative charge on plasma protein, the anion gap is reduced in hypoproteinemic states but is never less than 5 mEq/L. Some examples in the use of these relationships follow.

1. The laboratory reports the following values: sodium 120, chloride 95, bicarbonate 25 mEq/L. In this case the anion gap is 0, which is a physiological impossibility. Hence, one or more of the values reported is in error.

2. A patient reportedly has the following values: sodium 130, chloride 100, bicarbonate 20 mEq/L. In this case the anion gap is 10 mEq/L. Later the same day, the laboratory reports: sodium 140, chloride 100, bicarbonate 14 mEq/L, making the anion gap 26 mEq/L. In the absence of lactic acidosis or ketoacidosis, a 16 mEq/L increase in the anion gap in such a short period of time is unlikely; therefore, the values are suspect and should be remeasured.

When using either plasma sodium or freezing-point depression to measure plasma osmolality, certain precautions are required in the interpretation of the reported results. In the case of plasma osmolality, elevations due to urea should be disregarded, since this metabolite is distributed in the total body water and does not influence shifts of water between the intracellular and extracellular space. Changes in plasma os-molality due to increases in urea (reported from the laboratory as blood urea nitrogen or BUN) can be estimated as follows:

$$\frac{\Delta BUN \ (mg/100 \ ml)}{3} = \Delta Posm \ (mOsm/kg)$$

In the case of plasma sodium, acute elevation of extracellular solutes such as glucose or mannitol may cause hyponatremia due to shifts of water from the ICF to the ECF with dilution of the ECF sodium concen-tration. Thus, the plasma sodium concentration in this instance does not accurately reflect body osmolality or water requirements. Compensation for the depression of plasma sodium can be approximated by adding 2 mEq/L to the measured plasma sodium for each 100 mg/100 ml of blood glucose (or mannitol) elevation above normal.

Although shifts of water between the ICF and ECF are noted with *acute* elevations of blood glucose, this is not seen in the stable diabetic with *chronic* hyperglycemia. In this latter instance, the plasma sodium concentration is within the normal range and the elevation of blood glucose is reflected as an increase in plasma osmolality.

Water Depletion.   Water depletion (Figure 4–6) is defined as an increase in plasma osmolality or sodium and infers a decrease in cell water. However, it is important to understand that when a patient complains of thirst in the absence of hemorrhage or saline depletion and has a high urine osmolality or specific gravity, a diagnosis of water deple-tion can be made even if the plasma sodium is below 145 mEq/L (Posm <290 mOsm/kg), and the sicker the patient, the lower the plasma sodium may be with these signs present. In such instances it is wise to try to alleviate the patient's symptoms by giving extra water until such time as the plasma sodium reaches the 130 mEq/L range (Posm = 260 mOsm/kg). If thirst still persists, it is probably unwise to produce further water excess in order to relieve the symptoms, although there may be rare instances where this risk is worth taking to satisfy the comfort of the patient.

Water depletion, with the plasma sodium concentration rising above 145 mEq/L (Posm >290 mOsm/kg), usually develops in the settings noted in Table 4–2.

Severe depletion (plasma sodium > 160 mEq/L or Posm > 320 mOsm/kg) is most often seen where a defect of renal function is present, prolonged inadequate water intake has been present, the patient has sus-tained a large skin burn and water losses through this route are exces-sive, or renal concentrating capacity is impaired.

Physical signs are usually absent except in the more severe cases where the skin may become doughy and the patient irritable and depressed. The hematocrit does not increase in water depletion because there is a proportional loss of fluid from red cells and plasma. The only

Table 4-2. Causes of water depletion.

I. Primary water depletion (normal renal function)
  A. Inadequate intake
    1. Coma, general anesthesia
    2. Mental obtundation
  B. Excessive losses
    1. Skin: sweating, burns
    2. Gastrointestinal: vomiting, diarrhea, bowel drainage or fistula
  C. Reset of osmoregulatory center (rare)
    1. Idiopathic
    2. Brain lesion: hydrocephalus, tumor
II. Functional renal impairment
  A. Concentrating defect
    1. Diabetes insipidus
    2. Nephrogenic diabetes insipidus
    3. Hypokalemic nephropathy
    4. Hypercalcemic nephropathy
  B. Osmotic diuresis
    1. Glucose
    2. Mannitol
    3. Urea (including urea endogenously produced from high-protein tube feedings)

criterion needed for the diagnosis is an elevated plasma osmolality or sodium concentration.

The degree of elevation of Posm or plasma sodium concentration measures the magnitude of water depletion, and one does not need to further quantitate the deficit. The treatment is to give the basic allowance plus additional water for correction. *One ordinarily gives, at most, an extra liter of electrolyte-free water daily.* To infants one gives an additional 10 to 20 ml/kg daily. Too rapid correction of water depletion, especially in infants, may cause convulsions.

Water Excess.   Water excess (Figure 4–6) is defined as a decrease

Table 4-3. Causes of water excess.

I. Functional renal impairment without edema
  A. Extracellular volume depletion
  B. Primary adrenal insufficiency
  C. Primary inappropriate secretion of ADH
II. Functional renal impairment with edema
  A. Congestive heart failure
  B. Cirrhosis of the liver
  C. Nephrotic syndrome
III. Renal disease
  A. Acute renal failure with oliguria
  B. Chronic renal failure
IV. Excessive water intake with normal renal function
  A. Compulsive water drinking
  B. Iatrogenic: intravenous infusions, prostatic surgery with absorption of bladder fluid via the prostatic venous bed, etc.

in osmolality and infers an increase in cell water. With the one exception noted in Table 4–3, there is always a defect in the renal handling of water.

Signs and symptoms of hyponatremia are often absent; but when present they are those of diffuse cerebral dysfunction. Beginning with mental confusion, these symptoms progress in severity to muscle twitching, vomiting, delirium, and finally convulsions, coma, and death. Severity of symptoms depends more on the rate of lowering of osmolality than on the absolute level. Treatment consists of restricting water intake, which will slowly increase body osmolality and is adequate therapy in the majority of cases. To avoid the dangers of circulatory overload and saline excess, administration of hypertonic sodium solutions in the treatment of hyponatremia should be reserved for the emergency treatment of severe water excess producing mental obtundation or convulsions.

The extent to which body osmolality should be raised by treatment is not clear. Usually a plasma sodium level above 130 mEq/L (Posm >260 mOsm/kg) seems a reasonable goal. However, some severely ill patients, when water is restricted, will develop thirst and oliguria while still hyponatremic. A few of these patients appear to actively regulate water balance in order to maintain hyposmolality. In such patients, it is not clear which is worse, hyponatremia or thirst and oliguria. Usually, there is no elevation of plasma creatinine or BUN and there is little evidence that oliguria is harmful, although the thirst can cause great discomfort. On the other hand, the hyponatremia is usually symptomless.

Combined disorders (Table 4–4) present no special problems in either diagnosis or treatment, since each part of the disorder is diag-

Table 4–4. Possible disturbances of sodium and water balance in a 70 kg patient.

CONDITION	ECF (L)	PLASMA SODIUM (mEq/L)	CHANGE IN ECF (L)	COMMENT
1. Normal	15	140	0	
2. ECF depletion	8	140	−7	Caused by GI loss
	7.5	150	−7.5	of sodium and water
a. With water depletion				GI loss without water ingestion; osmotic diuresis
b. With water excess	9	120	−6	Renal defect in water excretion plus water ingestion
3. ECF excess	22	140	7	Only clinical evidence is edema
a. With water depletion	20	150	5	Water restriction plus edema
b. With water excess	24	120	9	Used to be called low-salt syndrome

nosed and treated separately. Two frequently encountered disorders warrant special comment.

Saline Depletion and Water Excess.   In order to become saline depleted, a patient must usually lose sodium by excessive sweating or from the gastrointestinal tract, since renal salt wasting is rare. Large ECF losses cause oliguria due to hypovolemia, which causes decreased renal blood flow and increased ADH secretion, both factors reducing renal water excretion. However, the patient can become hyponatremic *only* if he has access to enough exogenous water to make his free water intake greater than his losses. Thus, the low plasma sodium level sometimes seen in saline depletion (formerly used as a diagnostic criterion for saline depletion) actually represents a superimposed water excess. Even though the extracellular space is contracted, *the cells are swollen.*

The fact that a low plasma sodium is found in many patients with saline depletion has resulted in a great confusion regarding the interpretation of this value. Although it would seem logical to relate plasma sodium to sodium need, the relationship gives erroneous information most of the time. It is reasonable to raise the question of saline depletion in a patient with a low plasma sodium level, but it is essential that the issue be decided on other grounds. The low plasma sodium must be regarded only as evidence of water excess, one cause of which is saline depletion. Since there are numerous causes of water excess, the diagnosis of saline depletion must depend on the criteria discussed previously and not on the plasma sodium level.

Saline Excess and Water Excess.   The approach to sodium and water therapy developed in this chapter greatly simplifies the management of the confusing and poorly understood group of edematous patients who have in common the problem of hyponatremia. Because of the underlying mechanism, the fluid-electrolyte problem is managed by the usual treatment for sodium excess and water excess, namely, restriction of both sodium and water. In general, hypertonic sodium solutions have no place in the treatment. The question of what level of osmolality is reasonable for severely ill patients cannot be answered categorically because the pathogenesis of the water excess that develops in many severely ill patients is the most poorly understood aspect of fluid balance.

For a variety of complex reasons, many critically ill adult patients develop water excess and saline excess. In such patients the "osmostat" appears to be set at a lower level, and the patient appears to be regulating water balance to maintain a certain degree of hyposmolality. Regardless of the name attached, "hyponatremia of severe illness," "chronic dilutional hyponatremia," or others, the osmolar disturbance is best corrected by restricting water.

In general, edematous patients develop hyponatremia as the underlying disease process becomes more severe. These patients appear to be retaining water in an effort to maintain the hypervolemia of the edematous state. This syndrome has been given various names, the most common one being "low-salt syndrome." It might more properly have been called the "water retention syndrome." The development of water excess in an edematous patient indicates an almost hopeless prognosis unless the underlying disease can be successfully treated. Specifically, it means that the edema is becoming resistant to treatment and unless the underlying disorder, usually severe heart or liver failure, can be improved, the prognosis is very poor.

PHYSIOLOGICAL CONTROL OF POTASSIUM BALANCE

There are approximately 3500 mEq of potassium in body fluids and cells of a normal 70 kg person. Dietary intake amounts to about 100 mEq/day, with a comparable amount appearing in urine. Normal gastrointestinal losses in feces are small (5 to 10 mEq/day) and are not influenced by dietary manipulations. Urinary excretion is markedly influenced by dietary changes, but the renal response is not as rapid as that seen with changes in sodium ingestion. For example, it usually takes 10 to 15 days to see a significant reduction in urinary potassium excretion when a potassium deficient diet is taken; even then renal conservation is not complete, with 5 to 10 mEq/day being lost in the urine. Thus, an inadequate dietary intake may, even with normal gastrointestinal function, be the precursor of body potassium depletion due to renal losses.

Of the total body potassium, only about 70 mEq or 2 per cent of this total body potassium is in the extracellular space. The remainder is contained within the cell mass, about 70 per cent of it in skeletal muscle. Thus, it follows that the cell mass, and especially the muscle mass, determines the normal body potassium content.

If the *potassium capacity* is defined as being equal to the *total body potassium content at a time of normal potassium metabolism,* then the potassium capacity must be directly proportional to the cell mass or the muscle mass. The potassium capacity is related to the negatively charged intracellular anions which match the positively charged potassium. These anions are derived from the large amount of organic phosphate and from negatively charged protein groups, or from a combination of both. It would be expected, therefore, that factors affecting intracellular metabolism would produce changes in potassium capacity. For example, the cellular uptake of glucose is associated with a fall in plasma potassium concentration due to a concomitant intracellular transport of potassium. Protein anabolism is also associated with cellular uptake of potassium and, on the other hand, the rapid protein catabolism associated with trauma, infection, and tissue ischemia decreases capacity and may produce elevations of plasma potassium if renal function is impaired.

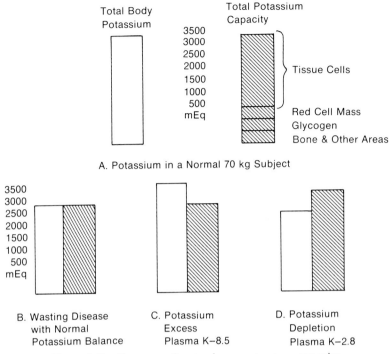

A. Potassium in a Normal 70 kg Subject

B. Wasting Disease
with Normal
Potassium Balance

C. Potassium
Excess
Plasma K—8.5

D. Potassium
Depletion
Plasma K—2.8

Figure 4–8.   Patterns of potassium content vs. capacity.

Obviously, the potassium capacity will vary greatly in different individuals and even in the same individual. Consider the following: a 70 kg individual may have a potassium capacity of 3500 mEq, but after a severe attack of paralytic poliomyelitis will have, due to protein catabolism and muscle wasting, a potassium capacity of, say, 1500 mEq and yet be in normal potassium balance because his total body potassium is also 1500 mEq.

By definition, potassium balance is normal when the total body potassium equals potassium capacity (Figure 4–8). Disturbances of potassium balance are defined in terms of this relationship. Potassium depletion is present whenever total body potassium is less than potassium capacity (Figure 4–8D). Potassium excess exists whenever total body potassium is greater than potassium capacity (Figure 4–8C). It is apparent that consideration must be given to changes in potassium capacity as well as changes in total body potassium. In fact, under certain circumstances, changes in potassium capacity are dominant in the genesis of potassium disorders. For example, in a patient with renal shutdown, potassium capacity decreases as muscle tissue is catabolized; potassium excess with high plasma potassium results because total body potassium remains constant due to kidney failure.

In order to diagnose and treat disturbances of potassium balance, criteria must be used which reliably reflect the relationship between total body potassium and potassium capacity. Fortunately, the plasma potassium reflects changes in this relationship, falling with potassium depletion and rising with potassium excess, thus serving as a useful guide to the potassium needs of the patient. The normal range of plasma potassium is 3.3 to 4.7 mEq/L, with a mean of 4.0 mEq/L.

Since the resting transmembrane electrical potential is caused by the ratio of intracellular to extracellular $[K^+]$, disorders of potassium metabolism change this ratio and induce changes in membrane potential. The clinical signs and symptoms related to the muscular, nervous, and cardiac systems in patients with severe hypokalemia and hyperkalemia are, in part, due to changes in cellular membrane polarization.

The following case examples clarify these principles.

Case 1.   A 70 kg man undergoes an extensive surgical procedure followed by a long period of infection with marked wasting. At the end of this period, measurements of potassium metabolism are compared with initial values. It is noted that his plasma potassium level is still normal. He has no symptoms of potassium depletion, and his electrocardiogram is normal. A piece of muscle taken for tissue analysis reveals a normal amount of potassium. Yet, balance studies carried on during the illness reveal a loss of half of the total body potassium. This large loss is accompanied by, and actually secondary to, a breakdown of about one-half of his living tissue mass, mostly muscle. Balance studies show a loss of 1 gm of nitrogen for every 3 mEq of potassium, the ratio of potassium to nitrogen in living tissue. Hence, he has had a 50% reduction in capacity. The net change from normal in this 70 kg man is diagrammed in Figure 4–8B. The total body potassium equals the potassium capacity, and the plasma potassium is 4.3 mEq/L, defining normal potassium metabolism.

Case 2.   A 70 kg woman suffers crushed injury to a leg and develops oliguric acute renal failure persisting for 12 days. During the first 5 days, the patient is maintained on parenteral 50% dextrose and fluid restriction. Acidosis is avoided by gastric suction, and some potassium is removed by this route. Despite this therapy, the rate of destruction of muscle from the injured leg markedly reduces the potassium capacity. Potassium excess ensues and the plasma potassium rises to 8.5 mEq/L on the fourth day. At this time, a muscle biopsy reveals a 15% increase in potassium, and the electrocardiogram shows signs of hyperkalemia. Thus, potassium excess has developed despite a slight negative potassium balance. The potassium capacity has decreased as a result of destruction of muscle cells in the crushed extremity, the breakdown of red blood cells, the general catabolism of tissue cells throughout the body, and possibly the depletion of glycogen stores in response to caloric deficit. The alterations from normal in this 70 kg patient are diagrammed in Figure 4–8C. Note that the total body potassium exceeds potassium capacity and plasma potassium is 8.5 mEq/L.

Case 3.   A 70 kg man on the sixth day after a gastrectomy developed a duodenal fistula. Gastrointestinal losses of over 2 liters per day are replaced with only dextrose in water and saline. Four days later blood electrolytes are normal except for a plasma potassium of 2.8 mEq/L. In this patient potassium capacity has decreased, and his glycogen stores and muscle protein are utilized for energy. However, total body potassium has decreased far more through fistula losses (Figure 4–8D). In the absence of an acid-base disorder, the low plasma potassium indicates significant potassium depletion.

Note the usefulness of the plasma potassium in these case examples. In Case 1 the total body potassium equals potassium capacity and the plasma potassium (4.3 mEq/L) is normal; the patient needs no added potassium despite the low total body potassium. In Case 2 the potassium capacity has been reduced more than the total body potassium, resulting in potassium excess, reflected by a plasma potassium of 8.5 mEq/L. In Case 3 the total body potassium is less than the potassium capacity, indicating potassium depletion with a plasma potassium of 2.8 mEq/L.

Effect of Acid-Base Imbalance on Plasma Potassium.   It has been shown both in experimental animals and in man that changes in extracellular pH will have an effect on the internal equilibrium between plasma potassium concentration and the potassium within cells. Acidosis *increases* and alkalosis *decreases* the plasma potassium level in relation to whatever content-capacity ratio exists at that given time. A possible explanation may be that changes in intracellular H^+ change the potassium capacity. The practical consequence of this observation is that the plasma potassium level can be considered to reflect the intracellular or total body potassium status only if there is no acid-base disorder present; or, at least, consideration must be made for existence of the acid-base abnormality. This means that in the presence of acidosis with a reduced blood pH, a normal plasma potassium signifies depletion and a low plasma level reflects severe depletion. When blood pH is high, a low plasma potassium level exists in the presence of normal intracellular stores. More accurate quantitation is discussed separately in the following section.

Quantitation of Potassium Disorders.   In the absence of acid-base disorders, estimation of the magnitude of the disorder from the plasma potassium level is fairly simple based on the principles that: (1) the magnitude of the disorders must be related to the size of the patient, or, more accurately, to the normal total body potassium (or capacity); and (2) the normal relationship between plasma level and intracellular state is semilogarithmic.

The quantitative relationship between plasma potassium and potassium depletion or excess has been described by studies which varied body potassium content under conditions of constant potassium capacity. The plasma potassium concentration on a logarithmic scale was found to be proportionate to the potassium content expressed as a percentage of potassium capacity. Potassium capacity was measured by radioactive potassium dilution at a time of normal potassium metabolism. This relation is shown in Figure 4–9.

Thus, the plasma potassium will define a potassium disorder as a per cent deviation from the potassium content-capacity ratio. If the total body potassium (or potassium capacity) were known, the milliequivalents of potassium depletion or excess could be calculated. A reasonable es-

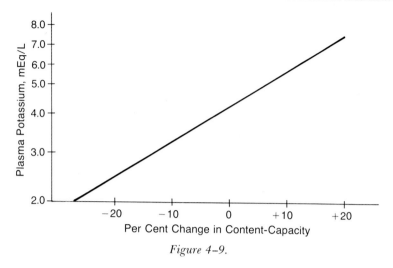

Figure 4–9.

timation of potassium capacity can be made from a simple estimation of the degree of wasting.

Estimation of Potassium Capacity

	Males	*Females*
Normal	45 mEq/kg	35 mEq/kg
Moderate wasting	32 mEq/kg	25 mEq/kg
Very marked wasting	23 mEq/kg	20 mEq/kg

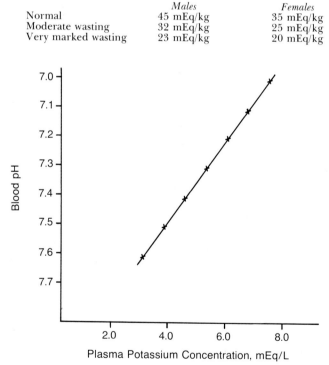

Figure 4–10. Effect of change in acid-base status on plasma potassium concentration with constant content-capacity.

Case Example. A patient is known to weigh 70 kg. He has lost 4 kg during his present illness and appears to be slightly wasted. The estimated potassium capacity might be 70 kg × 40 mEq/kg or 2800 mEq. From Figure 4–10, assuming no acid-base disorder, the depletion at a plasma potassium 2.8 mEq/L is about 13%, or 0.13 × 2800 to 3000 mEq or 360 mEq.

Quantitation of Effect of Acid-Base Disorders on the Plasma Potassium. A rough assessment of the influence of acid-base disorder on the relationship between the plasma potassium and intracellular potassium is necessary if plasma potassium is to be used as a guide to potassium therapy. This relationship is indicated in Figure 4–10. This depicts the influence of blood pH on plasma potassium with no change in body potassium stores. It can be seen that each 0.1 of a unit change in blood pH results in a change of about 0.7 mEq/L in the plasma potassium. Use of this information permits, if blood pH is known, an estimate of what the plasma potassium would be if no acid-base abnormality existed.

Case Example. A 40-year old woman enters the hospital with vomiting of three days duration. Plasma potassium is 3.0 mEq/L and blood pH is 7.60. Reference to Figure 4–10 shows that this is about what would be expected if there were no potassium disorders; that is, plasma potassium would be corrected to 4.5 mEq/L if the alkalosis were corrected to a blood pH of 7.40.

Quantitation of Potassium Disorders in the Presence of an Acid-Base Disturbance. A composite plot of the effect of a combination of potassium imbalances and acid-base disturbance on plasma potassium

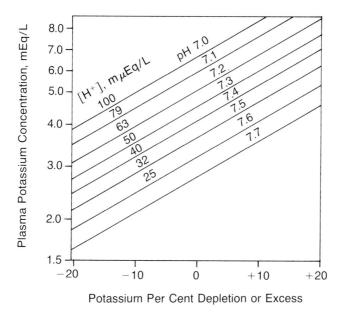

Figure 4–11. The relationship between plasma potassium concentration, blood pH and per cent change in content-capacity.

concentration can be made (Figure 4–11). If blood pH is measured, the plasma potassium can be corrected so as to reflect the magnitude of potassium disorder. Then by estimation of potassium capacity a general estimation of the magnitude of excess or depletion can be derived.

Case Example. A semi-comatose, elderly alcoholic man was brought to the hospital. He had been found in a downtown hotel and the only history was that of an old ulcer and recent vomiting. Plasma bicarbonate was 48, potassium was 2.2, and the blood pH was 7.58. Correction of plasma potassium for alkalosis revealed a corrected value of 2.8. This reflects a depletion of 16%. Since he was a small, wasted man, his total body potassium (or capacity) was estimated as 2000 mEq. Therefore, his depletion was 0.16 × 2000 or about 320 mEq.

DISTURBANCES OF POTASSIUM BALANCE

Potassium Depletion.   This is defined as a total body potassium less than the potassium capacity. Depletion may be recognized by *historical* circumstances leading to a negative balance, such as poor dietary intake or excessive gastrointestinal or renal losses. Diarrhea may lead to depletion because of the loss of large volumes of relatively potassium-rich fluid (20 to 40 mEq/L). Excessive urinary loss of potassium is seen post-operatively and with other stressful conditions with high adrenocorticoid output. Renal potassium loss is also increased in metabolic alkalosis and with diuretic and adrenocorticoid therapy. It is seldom possible to diagnose potassium depletion on the basis of history alone, because in sick patients the loss of potassium capacity due to tissue catabolism often keeps pace with potassium losses.

The *symptoms and signs* of potassium depletion usually do not appear until deficiency is marked. Symptoms consist of apathy, weakness, paresthesias, and tetany. Irregularities of cardiac rhythm may develop. With far advanced deficiency a flaccid paralysis may occur. The cranial nerves are rarely involved, but the muscles of respiration may be so weakened that the patient has to be mechanically ventilated. Potassium depletion predisposes to digitalis intoxication, a condition which always demands a measurement of plasma potassium.

The *plasma potassium level* is the most valuable aid in the diagnosis of potassium depletion. Diagnosis of potassium disturbances before they become severe is dependent upon abnormalities of the plasma level, a rather sensitive index, as shown in Figure 4–9.

The presence of *metabolic alkalosis* should always raise the question of potassium depletion, since gastrointestinal or renal loss of potassium, or both, are commonly associated with diseases producing this acid-base disorder. Despite this frequent association of potassium depletion and alkalosis, each condition does occur separately.

Changes in the *electrocardiogram* are not pathognomonic of potassium depletion but may be highly suggestive. Potassium depletion is characterized by a sagging of the ST segments, depression of the T waves, and elevation of the U waves. The QT interval appears to be prolonged only because the QU interval is mistakenly measured as the QT interval.

Renal concentrating ability is impaired and tubular injury occurs in patients with chronic potassium depletion. This may result in a polyuric state with renal wastage of water.

In summary, potassium depletion may be suggested by (1) recognition of causative events, (2) electrocardiographic changes, or (3) symptoms and signs. A low plasma potassium is confirmatory.

Prevention and Treatment of Potassium Depletion. Because large changes in total body potassium must occur before clinically significant depletion develops, it is relatively easy to prevent potassium depletion by careful attention to maintenance therapy. Great care in potassium administration is indicated in cases of possible renal shutdown, where there is always a threat of potassium excess.

The potassium given in excess of the basic allowance constitutes *corrective therapy.* As long as a large potassium depletion exists, there is little danger in the administration of as much as 20 to 30 mEq/hr, as potassium rapidly enters the cells and significantly elevated plasma levels are not seen.

However, the plasma potassium is more and more easily increased as normal potassium balance is approached. For this reason, it is wise never to attempt complete correction of potassium depletion in one day. A 30 to 50 per cent correction (but not exceeding 240 mEq) is recommended for one 24-hour period, with daily re-evaluation in most cases.

By distributing potassium dosage evenly in the fluids being administered, it is usually possible to keep potassium concentrations below 40 mEq/L in parenteral fluids. Occasionally, in cases of very severe depletion, it is necessary to use higher potassium concentrations, in which case careful control of the rate of infusion is mandatory to avoid any possibility of very rapid infusion leading to a high plasma potassium concentration and cardiac standstill. Oral administration of potassium-rich food or potassium salts is possible in cases not requiring parenteral fluids.

When potassium depletion and extracellular alkalosis co-exist, it is not necessary to decide which factor is the primary problem since potassium chloride is good treatment for both conditions. The chloride stays in the extracellular fluid, while the potassium may either enter cells if there is potassium depletion or be excreted in the urine in place of hydrogen.

Although oliguria is usually a contraindication to potassium therapy, uremia is not. The uremic patient often has a relatively high and fixed potassium loss, and therapy must be guided by serial measurements of the plasma potassium.

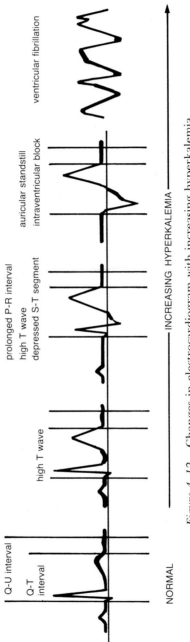

Figure 4–12.   Changes in electrocardiogram with increasing hyperkalemia.

Potassium Excess. This is defined as a total body potassium greater than the potassium capacity (Figure 4–8). Since normal kidneys rapidly excrete potassium loads, potassium excess is nearly always associated with oliguric renal failure and is usually associated with a decrease in potassium capacity. Potassium excess is especially prone to occur with a *historical* setting of oliguria accompanied by extensive tissue destruction, as with crush injury or in adrenocortical insufficiency where tubular secretion is impaired.

Symptoms and signs of potassium excess are usually non-existent. However, occasionally a patient will develop weakness and even a flaccid type of paralysis which is indistinguishable from that seen with hypokalemia.

Hyperkalemia is associated with electrocardiographic changes, but correlation is only fair. However, electrocardiographic changes precede hyperkalemic cardiac arrest and are the best index of approaching toxicity. Changes begin with tenting of T waves (Figure 4–12) and are followed by heightened T waves, QRS spreading, atrial arrest, and finally a sine wave heralding imminent cardiac arrest.

Hyperkalemia in states of potassium excess may be markedly aggravated by a reduction in blood pH (Figure 4–10). With a marked acidosis, a plasma potassium of 6 to 7 mEq/L may reflect normal intracellular stores, or a normal plasma potassium may reflect depleted stores.

The treatment of potassium excess is essentially the treatment of hyperkalemia. Cardiac toxicity roughly parallels the hyperkalemia whether elevation of the plasma level is secondary to intracellular potassium excess, to low blood pH, or to both. The aim of emergency treatment is two-fold: to combat the cardiac toxicity and to increase removal of excess potassium from the body. The abnormal electrophysiology associated with hyperkalemia (Figure 4–12) can be quickly reversed by an infusion of calcium gluconate; however, the effect is temporary, lasting only a few hours. A shifting of potassium into cells by correcting a low blood pH and infusing hypertonic (10 to 20%) glucose solution is helpful. If renal function can be improved by correction of saline depletion, this should be done. Otherwise, removal of excess potassium can be accomplished by cation exchange resins (orally or by colonic lavage) or by dialysis procedures.

DISORDERS OF ACID-BASE BALANCE

Acids, Bases, Buffers, and Hydrogen Ion Concentration. An *acid* is a molecule or ion that can give up hydrogen ions (protons). A *base* is a substance that can accept or bind hydrogen ions. Combinations of weak acids and strong bases are called *buffer systems* because they resist changes in hydrogen ion concentration by binding and releasing hydrogen ions.

The first line of defense against hydrogen ion change in the body is accomplished by the body buffers, which include the carbonic acid-bicarbonate system, as well as the proteins contained in extracellular fluid and body tissues in general. In addition to this "chemical" buffering, "physiological" buffering takes place through the excretion of hydrogen ions by the kidneys and carbonic acid by the lungs.

The acid-base status of the body is best expressed in terms of the concentration of hydrogen ion and body buffers. Because of theoretical and traditional reasons, pH, the negative logarithm of hydrogen ion concentration, is commonly used in biochemistry, physiology, and medicine. The pH system is a convenient expression since the range of hydrogen ion concentration in the body varies from 100 mEq/L (pH 1) in gastric fluid to 0.00001 mEq/L (pH 8) in pancreatic fluid. At the normal pH of 7.4, the blood and extracellular fluid contain 0.00004 mEq/L of hydrogen ion, or 40 nanoequivalents per liter (nEq/L). In disease states pH variations compatible with life may range from 6.9 to 7.6; thus, a five-fold variation of concentration is still compatible with life.

The Henderson-Hasselbalch Equation. Although other body buffer systems are quantitatively more important, the acid-base status can be assessed by measuring changes in the carbonic acid-bicarbonate system. In order to understand and evaluate changes in this buffer system, it is essential to be familiar with the Henderson-Hasselbalch equation and to appreciate its physiologic significance. This equation,

$$pH = 6.1 + \log \frac{[HCO_3^-]}{\alpha \cdot P_{CO_2}} \left(\text{from } pH = pK + \log \frac{[HCO_3^-]}{[H_2CO_3]} \right)$$

is derived by applying the Law of Mass Action to the reactions of the carbonic acid system:

$$CO_2 + H_2O \rightleftarrows H_2CO_3 \rightleftarrows H^+ + HCO_3^-$$

The constant 6.1 is pK, the first dissociation constant of carbonic acid at 37° C, plus a fudge factor to correct for the ionic strength of solution; α is a constant (0.031) which converts P_{CO_2} in mm Hg to $[H_2CO_3]$ in mM/L at 37°.

This equation demonstrates that the pH of the blood (or any other fluid compartment of the body) is uniquely determined by: (1) the *concentration of bicarbonate* in the blood, and (2) the *carbon dioxide tension* of the blood. Thus, a change in systemic pH *must* be accompanied by a change in one or both of these variables. The roles of various organs in regulating acid-base homeostasis can be summarized as follows: P_{CO_2} is regulated by the *lungs* acting under the direction of the *respiratory centers* in the brain; HCO_3^- is regulated by the *kidneys*. Consequently, disorders of acid-base balance may arise when the lungs, the respiratory centers, or the kidneys are damaged and cannot perform their homeostatic functions in a normal manner. In addition, disorders of acid-base balance occur when excessive amounts of acid or alkali are produced by, introduced into, or lost from the body.

Inspection of the Henderson-Hasselbalch equation shows that four *primary acid-base disturbances* can arise, corresponding to the various permutations of the $[HCO_3^-]/P_{CO_2}$ ratio.

1. *Metabolic acidosis* is due to a decrease in HCO_3^- or an increase in H^+. This disorder may arise from removal of HCO_3^- from the body in alkaline fluids or by addition of H^+ which reacts with HCO_3^- to form CO_2 and H_2O.

2. *Metabolic alkalosis*, similarly, is due to a rise in pH from accumulation of HCO_3^- or loss of H^+.

3. *Respiratory acidosis* is associated with a fall in pH due to an increase in P_{CO_2}.

4. *Respiratory alkalosis* is associated with a rise in pH from a decrease in P_{CO_2}.

From these definitions it might appear that a diagnosis of a metabolic acid-base abnormality could be made from knowledge of the plasma bicarbonate alone, or that a change in P_{CO_2} would indicate a respiratory abnormality. However, this is not the case because *each primary acid-base disturbance may produce a secondary compensatory reaction* which alters the P_{CO_2} in the case of a primary metabolic disturbance or the plasma bicarbonate in the case of a respiratory disturbance. The effect of such a compensatory reaction is to *reduce the deviation of systemic pH* from normal. For example, if the initial plasma bicarbonate is 24 mEq/L, the P_{CO_2} 40 mm Hg, and the pH 7.40, metabolic acidosis can theoretically occur with a fall in bicarbonate to 15 mEq/L, as illustrated below.

	$[HCO_3^-]$	P_{CO_2}	pH
uncompensated	15 mEq/L	40	7.20
partially compensated	15 mEq/L	30	7.32
completely compensated	15 mEq/L	23	7.44

In general, metabolic acid-base disturbances are associated with partial or no compensation. Respiratory disorders, when sustained, are associated with partial or even complete compensation.

Clinically the most frequently measured acid-base variable is the plasma bicarbonate. A low bicarbonate concentration may represent either: (1) a *metabolic acidosis*, (2) a *respiratory alkalosis*, or (3) a combination of both disorders. Consequently, a knowledge of the plasma bicarbonate concentration alone may indicate only the presence of an acid-base disturbance, but it does not distinguish the cause of the abnormality. In order to make an exact diagnosis, further information is necessary. This information may be provided by assessment of the clinical situation and by direct measurement of the blood pH or P_{CO_2}. In *most* instances where a single acid-base disturbance, whether uncompensated or compensated, is present, careful clinical evaluation together with the measured plasma bicarbonate and anion gap will lead to an accurate diagnosis. In other cases where the clinical situation is complex or where a combined acid-base disorder exists (such as a primary metabolic acidosis superimposed on a primary respiratory alkalosis) measurement of blood pH as well as bicarbonate or Pco_2 is necessary.

In attempting to relate a change in plasma bicarbonate to the amount of H^+ added to or removed from the body, it is important to keep in mind that the carbonic acid system is only one of the major body buffer systems. Other buffers provide a large reservoir for binding or releasing hydrogen ions in response to pH changes, but their activity is seldom obvious in clinical circumstances where only components of the carbonic acid system are measured. The role of non-carbonic acid buffer systems can be illustrated by considering the response to an acute respiratory alkalosis. When the Pco_2 is suddenly reduced by hyperventilation, an immediate fall in plasma bicarbonate occurs. Excretion of bicarbonate in the urine is negligible during the short time interval involved. What then has caused the loss of bicarbonate from the plasma? The answer is that as the pH rises in response to the decrease in Pco_2, hydrogen ions are released from hemoglobin and other non-carbonic acid buffers and react with bicarbonate, forming CO_2 and water. The magnitude of this process is sufficient to significantly lower the plasma bicarbonate concentration. The net result of this sequence is to reduce the rise in pH produced by the fall in Pco_2 and thus to provide some immediate partial compensation of the respiratory alkalosis. With time, if the diminished Pco_2 persists, renal bicarbonate reabsorption will decrease, resulting in increased bicarbonate excretion and providing an additional degree of compensation.

Acid-Base Homeostasis. Hydrogen ion differs from sodium and potassium and resembles water in its involvement in a complex of chemical reactions which constitute body metabolism. The actual intake of hydrogen ion in the diet is negligible compared with the amount which is generated in the oxidation of food and tissue. The combustion of carbohydrate and fat produces carbon dioxide, which dissolves in body water to give carbonic acid. Because the reaction is readily reversible, the lungs eliminate about 13,000 mEq/day of this *volatile acid* in the form of carbon dioxide. In the metabolism of protein, other acids are formed such as sulfuric, phosphoric, and certain organic acids, such as uric acid, which are not further metabolized by the body. The hydrogen ions produced in association with these processes, termed *metabolic* (or *nonvolatile*) hydrogen ions, are released from their anions into the body fluids where they are buffered. The normal person, on an average diet, produces 50 to 100 mEq of metabolic hydrogen ions per day, and this acid cannot be eliminated by the lungs but is dealt with by urinary excretion. If an increase or decrease in metabolic hydrogen ion production rate occurs, the kidney must adjust the rate of excretion of H^+ correspondingly; that is, the rate of NH_4^+ or titratable acid excretion or both must be changed. Sections in Chapter 2 described some of the mechanisms involved in titratable acid and NH_4^+ excretion. The manner in which these mechanisms can be used to vary H^+ excretion will be outlined.

There are four principal ways in which H^+ excretion in the urine can be increased (decreases in H^+ excretion can be produced by reversal of these mechanisms):

1. Urine pH can be lowered, leading to increases in both titratable acid and NH_4^+ excretion. Note that different mechanisms are involved in the effect of urine pH on these two forms of bound H^+. It is important to appreciate that in order to achieve a decrease in urine pH, a considerable increase in H^+ secretion must occur to provide the large numbers of hydrogen ions which bind to NH_3, phosphate, and other buffers as the urine pH falls as well as to provide the very small amount of free hydrogen ions involved in producing the change in pH.

2. Hydrogen ions can be retained in the blood, causing a systemic metabolic acidosis to develop, which stimulates NH_3 formation from glutamine in the kidney. The resulting increase in the partial pressure of ammonia in the kidney leads to increased NH_4^+ excretion. During systemic acidosis some hydrogen ions are also removed from the circulation by buffering in bone; thus, systemic acidosis enhances H^+ removal by both a renal and a non-renal route.

3. An increased rate of buffer excretion will lead to increased titratable acid excretion. If, for example, phosphate excretion increases, then hydrogen ion secretion will increase, resulting in increased titratable acid formation. However, unless there is an accompanying increase in phosphate production rate or intake, increased phosphate excretion will eventually result in phosphate depletion, which limits the value of this type of response for use in regulating H^+ excretion.

4. The partial pressure of NH_3 can be elevated by increasing the rate of entry of ammonium into the kidney by a higher arterial ammonium concentration or by providing more glutamine in the blood as substrate for intrarenal ammonia formation.

The first two of the above responses, decrease in urine pH and stimulation of renal NH_3 production by systemic acidosis, are both determined by alterations in intrarenal function and are the most important mechanisms available for regulating H^+ excretion by the kidney. The latter two responses, increase in buffer excretion or in arterial ammonium or glutamine, are the result of extrarenal changes which are influenced only slightly by the kidney; however, when such changes coexist with a need for increased H^+ excretion, the kidney can take advantage of them to assist in regulation of acid-base balance.

Responses to Ammonium Chloride Acidosis.   In the treatment of metabolic alkalosis, ammonium chloride or hydrochloric acid (in the form of lysine or arginine monohydrochloride) are occasionally given. The metabolic response to such treatment is instructive in understanding acid-base homeostasis, and will be described.

When ammonium chloride is administered, the NH_4^+ is converted by the liver to urea and other nitrogenous products, releasing H^+ and in effect adding hydrochloric acid to the body fluids. The hydrogen ions added to the blood react with HCO_3^-, forming H_2CO_3 and then CO_2, which is removed by ventilation resulting in a fall in HCO_3^-. A mild metabolic acidosis is thus produced which initially stimulates a fall in urine pH and, as must occur, associated increases in titratable acid and NH_4^+ excretion. These changes increase H^+, but not sufficiently to alleviate the acidosis. If the ammonium chloride load is continued over a period of several days, the persistent acidosis stimulates renal NH_3 production from glutamine and thus increases the renal NH_3 - NH_4^+ pool and NH_4^+ excretion. Some bone buffering of H^+ also occurs, reducing the amount of H^+ which the kidney must excrete to maintain homeostasis. As increasing amounts of NH_4^+ appear in the urine, the acidosis diminishes somewhat in severity and urine pH rises toward but not to the control level; titratable acid excretion falls in response to this increase in pH. After several days, a steady state of metabolic acidosis is achieved which must persist in order to maintain bone buffering and a high level of renal NH_3 production. Urine pH in this state is a little below normal and titratable acid excretion is a little above normal; NH_4^+ excretion is greatly increased, up to 5 or 6 times normal. At this time, the increased H^+ production rate will be balanced by H^+ removal through bone buffering and increased NH_4^+ excretion.

Outline of Clinical Disturbances of Acid-Base Balance

Metabolic acidosis.   This may arise from:

1. Excess of organic acid
   *a. diabetic ketoacidosis
   *b. lactic acidosis
   *c. salicylate, paraldehyde, methanol intoxication

2. Excess of inorganic acid
   a. NH₄Cl administration
   b. ureterosigmoidostomy

3. Impaired renal excretion
   *a. acute (oliguric) renal failure
   *b. chronic renal failure
   c. renal tubular acidosis (distal or proximal)

    4. Abnormal loss of bicarbonate
       a. GI: diarrhea, intestinal intubation and suction
       b. Renal: acetazolamide (Diamox) therapy

Estimation of the anion gap is clinically useful in diagnosing a metabolic acidosis. Those disorders associated with metabolic acidosis and an elevated anion gap are noted above with an asterisk. The increased anion gap is due to an excessive anion concentration associated with organic or inorganic acidosis.

Compensation. Chronic metabolic acidosis is usually partially compensated due to stimulation of respiratory activity by the fall in systemic pH. The degree of compensation which typically exists is seen in Figure 4–13.

Metabolic alkalosis. Sustained metabolic alkalosis can only occur in the presence of an increase in the renal threshold for bicarbonate reabsorption, thus permitting a high plasma bicarbonate to be maintained. Clinically this situation happens when chloride depletion which is out of proportion to sodium losses develops or when severe potassium depletion occurs. Such a circumstance may result from:

    1. Loss of acid (hydrochloric) by vomiting or gastric suction
    2. Loss of potassium chloride
       a. vomiting, gastric suction, diarrhea
       b. renal potassium wasting: diuretic therapy, primary or secondary aldosteronism, hyperadrenocorticism (Cushing's syndrome, ACTH therapy), potassium-losing nephropathy
    3. Excess base (bicarbonate, citrate, acetate)—effects usually transient

Compensation. Chronic metabolic alkalosis, unlike other acid-base disorders, is frequently uncompensated, especially when associated with potassium loss. Alveolar hypoventilation with an increase in PCO_2 does occur when exogenous alkali is given or when renal H^+ excretion is increased by ethacrynic acid or furosemide. The usual response to metabolic alkalosis is seen in Figure 4–13.

Respiratory acidosis. This disorder results from *hypoventilation* due to:

    1. Pulmonary disease: some alveoli are poorly perfused or substantial amounts of blood are shunted around the alveoli
    2. Limitation of respiratory movement: decreased elasticity of the lungs, weakened respiratory muscles or fixation of the ribs
    3. Decreased stimuli from respiratory centers: disease of respiratory centers or of pathway between CNS and lungs

Compensation. Increased PCO_2 enhances renal bicarbonate reabsorption with elevation of the plasma $[HCO_3^-]$. Because the stimulus for the change is PCO_2 rather than pH, complete compensation may occur, although partial compensation is usually encountered. The typical response, whether acute or chronic, is seen in Figure 4–13.

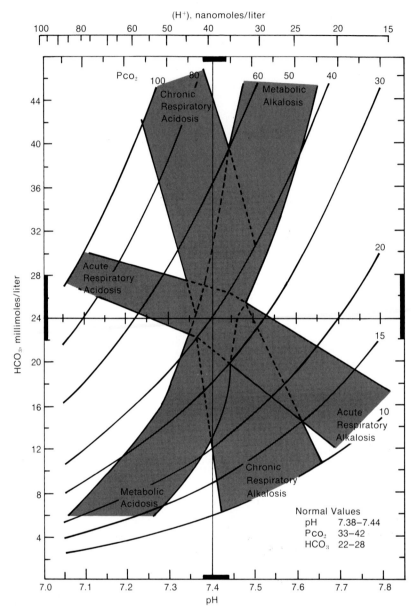

Figure 4–13. Nomogram of changes in blood pH, Pco_2, and bicarbonate concentration in various disease states.

Respiratory alkalosis. This disorder results from *hyperventilation,* usually neurogenic in origin, and is produced by a wide variety of causes such as fever, pain, anxiety, hypotension, epinephrine, and liver failure.
    Compensation. Chronic respiratory alkalosis decreases renal bicar-

bonate reabsorption through the reverse of the process that results in compensation for respiratory acidosis. The response to acute or chronic hyperventilation is seen in Figure 4–13.

Principles of Treatment of Metabolic Acid-Base Abnormalities

The first decision in determining the treatment of an acid-base disorder is to decide how harmful the abnormality in pH or Pco_2 is to the patient. Mild disorders, particularly metabolic acidosis and alkalosis, usually have no adverse effects and do not require correction. Severe abnormalities, on the other hand, may be life-threatening and demand immediate treatment.

The second step in treatment is to decide whether the underlying disease responsible for the acid-base disorder can be corrected. If so, the abnormality may be reversible without specific acid-base treatment. For example, many cases of diabetic acidosis can be treated with insulin and appropriate intravenous fluids without supplemental bicarbonate.

Specific Treatment. When specific therapy of a metabolic acid-base disturbance is required, complete correction of the abnormality is not necessary. As in the treatment of other fluid and electrolyte disorders, the goal is to correct the abnormality to a sufficient extent to eliminate its harmful effects on the patient, an objective which can usually be achieved by partial correction of the blood pH abnormality. The severity of the disturbance determines the rate at which reversal of the abnormality should be attempted and as improvement occurs, the rate of acid or alkali administration can be correspondingly tapered.

A compelling reason for avoiding too rapid correction of a metabolic acid-base disorder is related to the effect of such a correction on spinal fluid pH. The spinal fluid bicarbonate changes slowly in response to changes in plasma bicarbonate. For example, if a patient with a compensated metabolic acidosis (low HCO_3^- and low Pco_2) has his plasma bicarbonate rapidly restored to normal, the Pco_2 will quickly return to normal also. In the spinal fluid, the Pco_2 rises to normal because of rapid diffusion of CO_2 across the blood-brain barrier. However, spinal fluid bicarbonate does not equilibrate quickly with blood bicarbonate, and bicarbonate in the CSF remains low. The result is a return of blood pH to normal but an accentuation of the acidosis in the spinal fluid. The situation may result in a worsening of the clinical picture with development of coma and other neurologic signs.

Metabolic Acidosis. Only a crude guess at the magnitude of base deficit in metabolic acidosis can be made, and it is of limited value to try to quantitate the amount of alkali which must be added to body fluids to correct the acidosis. There are two reasons for this uncertainty. First, the buffer capacity of the body is not accurately known in an individual. Second, the rate of acid production varies widely in different situations leading to metabolic acidosis. For example, in methanol intoxication rapid infusion of bicarbonate may be necessary just to keep up with the rate of formic acid production; in acute renal failure, on the other hand, acid production may be limited to a normal rate of around 50 mEq/day and only small amounts of bicarbonate are required to maintain homeostasis. For these reasons, calculations of base deficit are inherently inaccurate and therapy based on the results will usually result in under- or over-shooting the normal acid-base state. And, to repeat, it is undesirable to attempt rapid correction of metabolic acidosis.

The obvious and direct approach to treating severe metabolic acidosis is to raise the plasma bicarbonate concentration by the administration of oral or intravenous sodium bicarbonate. In situations where rapid acid production is not present, the amount of bicarbonate necessary to correct the extracellular fluid deficit is a reasonable initial therapeutic maneuver and dosage can be estimated by multiplying the estimated ECF (liters) by the deficit in plasma bicarbonate:

$$ECF \times (24 - \text{measured plasma bicarbonate}) = \text{bicarbonate dosage (mEq)}$$

Such therapy will not totally correct the acid-base disturbance but will avoid the problems mentioned above. After bicarbonate administration, the acid-base status can be re-evaluated and additional treatment given as required.

In occasional cases of severe metabolic acidosis associated with advanced renal insufficiency, sodium bicarbonate administration is undesirable. In such patients, excretion of sodium is impaired and administration of a sodium salt may lead to over-expansion of the plasma volume, hypertension, and pulmonary edema. In place of bicarbonate administration, dialysis may be necessary to alleviate the metabolic acidosis.

In metabolic acidosis associated with stable chronic renal disease, the degree of pH aberration is small and plasma bicarbonate is usually above 15 mEq/L. This degree of acidosis occurs in patients with chronic renal failure; oral sodium bicarbonate or a mixture of sodium and potassium citrates (Shohl's solution) can be given. However, such patients frequently require low-sodium diets in order to treat their hypertension, and sodium administration may be contraindicated. In this situation, calcium carbonate is useful for treating acidosis instead of sodium bicarbonate.

Metabolic Alkalosis.   The pathogenesis of this acid-base disorder usually implies that a state of chloride depletion exists. Treatment with potassium and sodium chlorides will usually be sufficient to restore the renal bicarbonate threshold to normal and allow the homeostatic mechanisms of the body to correct the alkalosis. Severe potassium depletion by itself may result in metabolic alkalosis and, since chloride depletion is nearly always associated with some potassium loss, it is prudent to correct the chloride deficit in part with potassium chloride when potassium is not otherwise contraindicated. Occasionally the use of acetazolamide, ammonium chloride, or even hydrochloric acid may be required when severe metabolic alkalosis occurs in a complicated clinical setting. Ammonium toxicity and venous spasm produced by hydrochloric acid limit the usefulness of these agents.

Respiratory Disorders.   Treatment of respiratory acidosis, when indicated, requires improvement in ventilation to allow more rapid elimination of CO_2 from the body. This therapeutic goal is frequently difficult to achieve, especially in patients with chronic obstructive pulmonary disease. Careful treatment of the underlying respiratory disease is necessary and mechanically assisted ventilation is often required. Respiratory alkalosis is seldom severe or persistent and generally does not require treatment.

PATHOPHYSIOLOGY OF RENAL ACIDOSIS

By combining principles of homeostasis with a knowledge of renal acid-base physiology, the pathophysiology of various types of acidosis produced by impairment of renal function can be understood.

Reduction in Number of Functioning Nephrons

Acute Renal Failure.   In oliguric states resulting from tubular injury or severe glomerulonephritis, the ability of the kidneys to regulate acid excretion may be destroyed. This situation represents a failure of homeostatic regulation in which metabolic hydrogen ion production continues, but the mechanism for elimination is absent. Hydrogen ions produced by metabolism accumulate in the blood, producing progressive metabolic acidosis. The rate of development of the acidosis will depend on the rate of hydrogen ion production.

Chronic Renal Failure.   In advanced renal insufficiency a stable metabolic acidosis characteristically develops. The state of renal failure at which acidosis becomes apparent varies greatly from one patient to another. Most patients with a GFR of less than 20 ml/min have a diminished plasma bicarbonate, but acidosis may occur much earlier in the course of renal disease. Since the acidosis in this situation tends to be stable, we can conclude that it represents a homeostatic adaptation to the reduction in nephron mass. That is, the acidosis is essential in order to stimulate elimination of enough acid from the circulation each day to keep pace with acid production. The pathophysiology of this response can be outlined as follows:

1. The rate of acid production is determined by the diet. The amount and type of sulfo- and phospho-proteins ingested are the principal variables in acid production. Many patients with advanced renal failure are prescribed low protein diets, and therefore, in such individuals, *acid production is frequently diminished* compared to that found in subjects eating a normal diet.

2. Titratable acid excretion is often moderately diminished in patients with chronic renal failure. The amount of H^+ excreted in the form of titratable acid depends chiefly on: (a) the pH of the urine, and (b) the amount of phosphate excreted. Since most patients with chronic renal failure are able to acidify their urine to a normal degree, titratable acid excretion in this condition is limited chiefly by phosphate excretion, which in turn is determined by phosphate production rate. Like the H^+ production rate, phosphate production is reduced in advanced renal failure when a low protein diet is used in therapy.

3. Ammonium excretion is greatly reduced in chronic renal failure. Since most of the NH_4^+ in the urine is derived from NH_3 produced in the renal cortex, the amount of NH_4^+ excreted is diminished when nephron mass is reduced. In addition, the decrease in renal blood flow reduces delivery of arterial NH_4^+ to the kidney and the component of NH_4^+ in the urine which is derived from this source.

4. Total H^+ excretion in the form of titratable acid and NH_4^+ is insufficient to equal H^+ production. A state of metabolic acidosis therefore develops and results in two compensatory responses which permit the elimination of more H^+ from the circulation. First, the acidosis stimulates NH_3 production from glutamine in the kidney, increasing NH_4^+ excretion per nephron (*total* NH_4^+ excretion is still subnormal however). Second, balance studies have shown that acidosis promotes removal of some H^+ by a non-renal route, probably by bone buffering.

5. The development of acidosis will progress until H^+ production is balanced by the three processes for acid removal, titratable acid excretion, NH_4^+ excretion, and bone buffering. When this balance is achieved, the acidosis will stabilize, producing the persistent, mild chronic metabolic acidosis seen in chronic renal disease.

Renal Tubular Acidosis (RTA).   Two types of functional abnormalities occur in the kidney which lead to metabolic acidosis. In their pure form these disturbances occur with normal glomerular filtration rates, and the term RTA has been used to distinguish these disorders from the acidosis which develops when nephron mass is reduced. Renal tubular acidosis may be associated with renal stones or intrarenal calcification resulting eventually in renal failure. When this occurs, acidosis due to decreased nephron mass may be superimposed on renal tubular acidosis, producing a particularly severe acidotic state.

"Distal RTA."   In this form of RTA the primary functional abnormality is an inability to lower urine pH below about 6.0 regardless of the state of systemic acid-base balance or of other factors which normally stimulate urinary acidification. Thus, some poorly understood alteration in the cells of the collecting ducts impairs hydrogen ion secretion against a concentration gradient. Other aspects of renal acid-base metabolism, such as bicarbonate reabsorption in the proximal tubule and ammonium production from glutamine, are normal in this condition. Since the rate of both titratable acid excretion and ammonium excretion are determined in part by urine pH, patients with RTA and normal systemic acid-base balance will excrete decreased amounts of titratable acid and ammonium. Hydrogen ion production will, therefore, exceed H^+ excretion and acidosis will develop. Despite the acidosis, urine pH will remain at 6.0 and titratable acid excretion will also be fixed (unless extra phosphate is ingested). The acidosis will stimulate NH_3 formation from glutamine. Because urine pH remains high, much of the increased NH_3 production will leave the kidney in the renal vein but enough will reach the urine to increase total NH_4^+ excretion and to augment H^+ elimination. Thus the urine of a patient with distal RTA will show an increased NH_4^+ excretion when compared to a normal subject with the same urine pH. The systemic acidosis will also stimulate bone buffering of H^+, reducing the amount of acid which must be excreted by the kidneys in order to maintain homeostasis. These compensations will result in a new state of homeostasis in which metabolic acidosis is a necessary feature.

"Proximal RTA." In recent years another impairment of renal acidification has been described and has been termed *proximal tubular acidosis.* In this condition the reabsorptive threshold for bicarbonate in the proximal tubule is decreased so that bicarbonate ion spills over into the urine when the plasma bicarbonate concentration is normal. The result of this bicarbonate "leak" is to produce a subnormal steady state plasma bicarbonate. When this level of bicarbonate is reached, urine acidification will proceed normally and urine pH may be below 6.0, in contrast to distal RTA. The decreased plasma bicarbonate reflects the presence of a metabolic acidosis which results, as in the previous examples, in increased NH_3 production and in bone buffering. Fluctuations in urine pH in this disorder will regulate titratable acid and NH_4^+ excretion in response to changes in the rate of hydrogen ion production.

Treatment of Fluid Balance Disorders

Formulating the Daily Plan of Therapy. The approach to fluid and electrolyte therapy introduced in this section depends on the formulation of a daily plan of therapy. Before beginning to plan fluid therapy, it is necessary to know as much as possible about the patient and his fluid-electrolyte problems. The history often provides valuable information as to the type of fluid imbalance the patient has or is likely to develop. A patient with a history of congestive heart failure is likely to develop saline excess. A patient with an ulcer history who has been vomiting is likely to have saline and potassium depletion and metabolic alkalosis. In acute illness, a knowledge of weight loss, especially in infants, may give a rough approximation of the magnitude of fluid losses. A very careful history of stool, urine, and emesis is desirable. Reports of fever, changes in respiratory rate and the nature and amount of recent oral or parenteral intake are important.

Symptoms and physical signs may lack specificity, and both appear only with advanced disorders. In general, early recognition of a potential fluid balance problem should result in a plan of therapy which prevents the appearance of symptoms or signs.

Hematocrit and plasma electrolyte values are of great value in the diagnosis of fluid imbalance and must be obtained at the outset in every case of suspected imbalance. The determinations of plasma sodium, potassium, chloride, bicarbonate, glucose, and creatinine or BUN are now routinely available in most hospitals.

Measurement and recording of the details of the daily *intake and output* of fluid and electrolyte is a valuable aid in following day-to-day alterations in fluid balance and in making basic allowances. However, actual calculations of the daily water balance (the difference between the total intake and output) is to be *avoided* because the balance can be grossly inaccurate and bears little relation to the water needs of the patient. (Note that the fluid output total has been crossed out in the balance sheet in Table 4–5.)

On the other hand, in patients with very complex problems, determination of sodium or chloride balance can be a valuable aid in determination of saline needs. Serial determinations of *body weight* can also be used as a guide to saline need if body mass and osmolality are stable or appropriate corrections for changes are made.

Quantitative urine collections are usually obtainable in adults and older children, but they are ordinarily not performed in infants who are voiding well and making good progress, because of difficulties in accurate collection. If urine volumes need to be quantitated, it is important to employ one of the various devices designed to permit collections without catheterization if possible.

Table 4–5.   Intake–output record.
From 8 a.m. June 4 to 9 a.m. June 5. Equals 25 hr.

| INTAKE | | | | | OUTPUT | | | TOTAL | | |
VOL.		K$^+$	Na$^+$	Cl$^-$	VOL.		K$^+$	Na$^+$	Cl$^-$	pH
2000	10% D/S		300	300	400	Urine: Sugar: 0 Spg: 1.022			32	7.0
1000	10% D/W				1000	S & I		0	0	
	with KCl	80		80	2300	GI	23	230	230	5.0
3000	TOTALS	80	300	380	X	TOTALS			262	

Table 4–6.   Average daily basic allowances.

Loss	Water ML	Sodium mEQ	Chloride mEQ	Potassium mEQ
Urine	1500	50	90	40
Sensible & Insens.	1000	0	0	0
Gastrointestinal	Prev. vol. plus trend	equal or half Cl (see text)	100 mEq/L or measured	10 mEq/L

Using all available information about the patient, the plan of therapy can be formulated in two steps. First, the *basic allowance* is estimated for fluids and electrolytes. The basic allowance is the amount of fluid and electrolyte needed to replace anticipated gastrointestinal and sensible-insensible losses plus allowances for urine output which permit renal correction of imbalances. The second step in formulating a plan of therapy is making *correction allowances* for known abnormalities not corrected by the kidney or lungs. The total of basic and correction allowances becomes the amount of fluid and electrolyte to be given, or the *planned intake.*

Although the plan is formulated for the 24-hour period for convenience, it is often necessary to actually order fluids for only a few hours ahead by taking an appropriate fraction of the 24-hour amounts. In general, the sicker the patient or the larger his planned fluid intake, the shorter the therapeutic period should be.

Estimation of Basic Allowances.   The usual values for basic allowances in adults are shown in Table 4–6, and the proportion of these allowances for children over 12 kg in weight is shown in Table 4–7. Infants weighing less than 12 kg have problems peculiar to their age group and must have their therapy more closely tailored to their need.

The reasons for selecting these allowances for adults and older children and conditions under which they should be modified are based on physiological concepts discussed in the following sections.

Urine.   The basic allowance for urinary loss should be selected to provide the kidney with the best opportunity to help correct and maintain fluid and electrolyte balance. This allowance should represent values half-way between minimal and maximal excretion rates for that par-

Table 4–7.   Modification of allowances for children.

Weight KG	Per cent of Adult Allowances
15	50
25	75
45	100

ticular patient. The 1500 ml of water allowance is based on the assumption that the kidney of a sick patient can excrete as little as 500 ml and as much as 2500 ml of water in the event that the water administered does not match the need. Basic urinary allowances for sodium and potassium are arrived at by similar reasoning. For convenience, the basic allowance for chloride is taken as the sum of the cation allowance, and is not selected primarily to facilitate renal adjustment.

It is seldom necessary to change basic allowances for urine output. Occasionally, however, the kidney may lose its ability to regulate water balance or one of the electrolytes. Such a defect in renal regulation will be evident from the history or will become evident because of the abnormality it produces. To compensate for the defect, the urine allowance should be changed to fit the functional capacity of the kidney. For example, severely ill patients sometimes develop oliguria. This defect may cause the patient to develop water excess. A urine volume below 1500 ml in the presence of a low or falling plasma sodium level invariably points to a defect in the renal regulation of water and calls for appropriate change in the basic allowance for urine water. Another example of defective renal regulation is the presence of edema, which always indicates a large saline excess and calls for reduction to zero in the basic allowance for urinary sodium. In renal shutdown, basic urinary allowances are reduced to near zero.

Skin and Lungs.   Only when excessive sweating is anticipated should the allowances in Table 4–6 be altered. In such instances, the sensible-insensible loss may need to be increased by 500 to 1000 ml or up to several liters in hot humid climates.

Gastrointestinal Losses

Water.   An estimate of the volume of fluid to be lost through the GI tract of a patient during the therapeutic period under consideration is best arrived at by considering the losses during the period immediately preceding the current period. Thus, if a patient has been putting out 1500 ml of gastric fluid daily for several days, the chances are reasonably good that he will continue to do so. At least, this is the best basis for estimation of the output. If the output through the GI tract is increasing or decreasing, this trend should be considered. If there are no previous data even by history on which to base the estimate of output, then an educated guess must be made, as, for example, during the first 24-hour period following a gastric resection. Surgeons have learned from experience that the output through a gastric suction following gastric resection is usually between 500 and 1000 ml. No matter what figure is selected as the basic allowance for gastrointestinal losses, it is only an estimate subject to revision at any time during the therapeutic period, should the actual output change.

Sodium and Chloride.   The output of chloride in gastrointestinal fluid from the previous day's output can be measured or, in most instances, be assumed to be 100 mEq/L. The output of sodium will, for practical purposes, equal the output of chloride in all gastrointestinal fluids with a pH above 4. If the pH is 4 or below, consider the sodium output to be one-half the chloride output.

Potassium. Although the amount of potassium in gastrointestinal fluids can vary widely, for practical purposes an output allowance of 10 mEq/L is a reasonable figure to use.

Allowance for Correction of Imbalances. An orderly approach to the evaluation of fluid imbalances requires that the following question be answered. Does the patient have any imbalances detectable in these categories?

1. Water
2. Saline
3. Blood and Plasma
4. Acid-Base
5. Potassium

Thus, under "correction allowances" a line is provided for each of these categories, as shown in Table 4–8. Corrections can be either positive or negative. It is obvious that a negative correction cannot be larger than the basic allowance. Thus, in a patient with renal shutdown and severe water excess, if the basic allowance for water is 1000 ml, the maximum possible correction is minus 1000 ml.

Although the details regarding correction allowances are found in appropriate subsequent sections, the following general principles apply.

Water Requirements. The principles governing adjustment of water dosage are based on the assumption that the plasma osmolality as reflected in the plasma sodium level is an accurate and sensitive guide to the patient's water need. It is considered a desirable therapeutic goal to regulate *water intake* so as to maintain a plasma sodium above 130 mEq/L and below 145 mEq/L. If the plasma sodium concentration is outside these limits, appropriate corrections for water are made.

Saline Requirements. Estimates of the magnitude of alteration in extracellular volume make use of history and physical and laboratory findings. If there is doubt, the basic allowance for sodium should be given. When correction of a saline imbalance is made, the correction involves both electrolyte and water. For example, if a correction of plus 2 liters is decided upon, the correction would be: plus 2000 ml in the water column and plus 300 mEq in the sodium and chloride columns.

Blood and Plasma Requirements. Replacement is based on the assessment of the adequacy of the patient's blood volume as previously discussed and by determining on the basis of history, hematocrit, and plasma protein levels whether blood, plasma, or saline is required to increase blood volume.

Acid-Base Requirements. As discussed elsewhere, the history and physical and laboratory findings are used to establish the presence of an

Table 4–8. Fluid balance work sheet for daily fluid and electrolyte therapy

Date_____

Time_____

Patient_____ Age_____ Ward_____

From_____ to_____ Period No._____

Allowances

Basic Allowance

Source	Volume	Na	Cl	K
Est. S & I				
Urine				
G.I.				
Totals				

Correction Allowances

Water _____

Blood Volume_____

Saline _____

Acid-Base _____

Potassium _____

Combined Totals_____

Planned Intake:

Fluid Orders:

acid-base disturbance. Metabolic acidosis is prevented and treated by substituting bicarbonate, or an anion, such as lactate, which can be metabolized for the chloride usually given. Metabolic alkalosis is usually treated by administration of sodium, potassium, or ammonium chloride. Correction can be shown by adding or subtracting chloride or by adding columns for NH_4^+ or HCO_3^-.

Potassium. In general, potassium therapy is determined in large part by measurement of the plasma potassium, which gives a general estimate of the magnitude of the disorder. *It must be emphasized that any patient with azotemia or a daily urine volume below 500 ml should not receive potassium until hyperkalemia has been excluded.* At the same time, administration of the basic allowances of potassium as soon as it is safe to do so will prevent potassium depletion in the majority of patients.

Planning Treatment of Disturbances. Once a specific imbalance is diagnosed, correction allowances must be made. These allowances can be either positive or negative depending upon the type of imbalance. For example, with saline excess (edema), the correction allowance might be minus 2 liters of saline.

The problem of determining the exact magnitude of correction allowances is not difficult, provided the following general principles are adhered to:

1. Only a rough estimate of the magnitude of the disturbance is needed as a general guide to dosage. Determination of the exact dose needed for full correction of an abnormality is neither desirable nor possible.

2. The initial treatment of a disturbance should be most vigorous in the most severe disorders, but it should never aim at full correction during the first period. Remember that even stabilizing the situation by providing the basic allowance, and thus preventing progression of a disturbance, will often improve the patient. Furthermore, too rapid correction can produce new symptoms which may be more devastating than the original ones.

3. As treatment of an imbalance proceeds, and evidence of the disturbance becomes less definite, therapy should more nearly approach replacement of the basic allowance, thus allowing the patient's kidney the major role for the final stages of correction.

Translating the Plan of Therapy into a Fluid Order. The fluid order identifies each bottle by consecutive number from the beginning of treatment. It specifies the basic solutions required, lists the additives to be used in that solution, and gives an approximate infusion schedule. The fluid order is usually written for 24 hours ahead. In many instances, and especially when intake exceeds 3 liters, the fluid order must be evaluated once or twice during the 24-hour period.

Dextrose in water or saline is used to supply water, sodium, and chloride in the desired amounts. The problem of what dextrose concentration (5, 10, 20, or 50%) to use is a question of supplying calories versus sparing the veins. Five per cent dextrose is isosmotic to plasma, but higher concentrations are irritating and produce phlebitis. Whatever the choice, every solution given should contain at least 5% dextrose to supply needed calories.

Potassium should be divided equally among the bottles of administered fluid, since it is important that it be given slowly. Except for unusual circumstances, potassium should not be given faster than 20 mEq/hr because of the danger of producing hyperkalemia.

Route and Technique of Infusion. The subcutaneous route has few advantages and many disadvantages, and is not recommended. The intravenous route is safe provided the fluid is given slowly. Except for the early part of the treatment of profound acute disorders, intravenous fluids should always be given slowly — 500 ml an hour is the suggested rate. Much slower rates are required for hypertonic solutions.

If the patient requires an intake in excess of 4 liters, is extremely ill, or is receiving a large number of calories by vein, a 24-hour infusion is mandatory. This need not unduly bother the patient if a plastic needle or plastic intravenous catheter is used. However, the use of such apparatus involves a risk of phlebitis and infection and should not be left in a vein without daily inspection and removal to another site within 48 to 72 hours or sooner if inflammation is noted.

Chapter 5

DISEASES OF THE URINARY TRACT

The most dangerous ischuria is that in which the kidneys secrete no urine from the blood.

WILLIAM HEBERDEN (1710–1801)

As men draw near the common goal
Can anything be sadder
Than he who, master of his soul,
Is servant to his bladder?

ANONYMOUS
The Speculum, Melbourne, No. 140 (1938)

CONGENITAL ANOMALIES

The understanding of the major congenital abnormalities of the urinary system requires some background knowledge of embryology. Since a detailed treatment of embryology is beyond the scope of this syllabus, other references will be needed for further clarification. Congenital urinary abnormalities are important when they interfere with the function of the urinary system.

The most extreme abnormality is that of renal agenesis or complete absence of renal tissue. This is very rare (1 in 2700 *pediatric* autopsies), uniformly fatal, and primarily found in stillborn males.

Abnormalities of *size and number* of kidneys vary in occurrence and importance. A *solitary kidney* (unilateral renal agenesis) (Fig. 5–1, FSB–1) is seen in about one in 500 autopsies. Since it is asymptomatic, clinical discovery is usually a result of work-up for other disease processes. Single kidneys are usually enlarged (compensatory hypertrophy) since their functional requirement is doubled. When a kidney is removed, compensatory hypertrophy of the remaining kidney occurs in a patient at any time up to about 50 years of age. The etiologic mechanism is not well established, but apparently is humoral. The clinical importance of

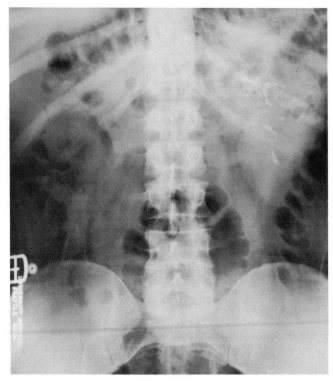

Figure 5–1 (FSB–1). Solitary kidney (unilateral renal agenesis). There is no functioning kidney seen on the patient's right and no renal shadow. Left kidney is markedly enlarged (5 vertebral bodies long, as compared with usual $3\frac{1}{2}$ vertebral bodies).

the solitary kidney is mainly that of recognition. Instances of removal of the single kidney for tumor, infection, trauma, cysts, or other reasons point out the ease with which such an error can be made if the possibility is not considered. *Supernumerary* (extra) kidneys do not present such a problem and are also extremely rare, though some 10% of all individuals have some degree of duplication in the renal pelvis. *Congenitally small* kidneys (renal hypoplasia) are also rare. Most instances of small kidney size are secondary to pyelonephritis, glomerulonephritis, or vascular disease.

Ectopic kidneys (Fig. 5–2, FSB–2) or abnormalities in the location of the kidney are somewhat less frequent than single kidneys. *Simple ectopia* is malposition of a normally lateralized kidney. The most frequent location is within the true pelvis. *Crossed ectopia* is a disturbance in lateralization in which the kidney is drained by a ureter which crosses the midline to empty into the bladder. There is no sex predilection. Because of abnormal location or abnormal rotation, the kidney is particularly susceptible to trauma or obstruction, with resultant infection or infarction. This

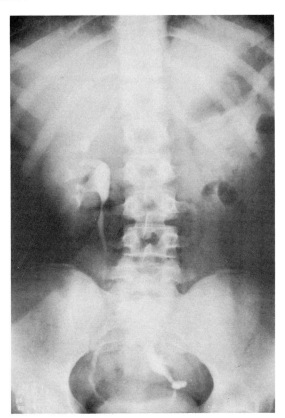

Figure 5-2 (FSB-2). Ectopic kidney. Left kidney seen in true pelvis. Right kidney is normal size.

abnormality is one of the few that do not have a logical embryological explanation. *Horseshoe kidneys* (Figure 5-3, FSB-3; Figure 5-4, FSB-4) occur with a frequency of approximately one per 400 to 700 live births. The most frequent site of fusion is the lower pole (90%). The kidney mass is usually fused anterior to the aorta and superior to its bifurcation. This abnormality has clinical significance because of the associated abnormalities of location and rotation. Since the kidney is fixed to its counterpart on the opposite side, it cannot rotate normally during development, thus leaving the renal pelvis anteriorly in the unrotated position. Such abnormal placement of the pelvis and course of the ureter (anterior over the isthmus of the horseshoe) predisposes to obstruction. A horseshoe kidney frequently has associated abnormalities in vascular supply, with multiple renal arteries arising from the aorta at levels from the superior mesenteric to the common iliac arteries.

    Significant anomalies of the collecting system (renal pelvis and ureter) are chiefly the result of improper branching of the ureteral bud or improper assimilation of the lower end of the ureter into the bladder. Probably the most common and minor defect is the partial division of the renal pelvis to form a bifid pelvis. This *duplication of the renal pelvis*

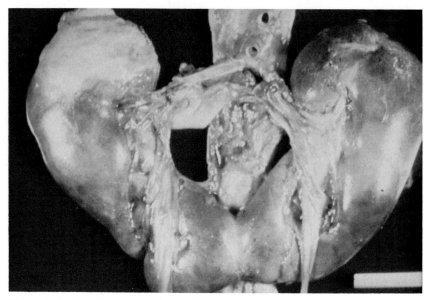

Figure 5-3 (FSB-3). Horseshoe kidney. Note the fusion at the lower pole and the anterior placement of the renal calyces. The ureters may be seen passing over the anterior surface of the isthmus.

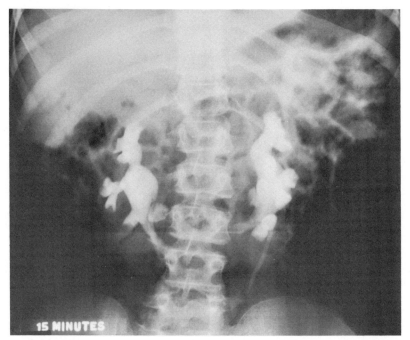

Figure 5-4 (FSB-4). Horeseshoe kidney. Note calyces pointing medially from the renal pelvis as a result of incomplete rotation; the long axes of the kidneys meet inferiorly (the lower poles are connected by the isthmus).

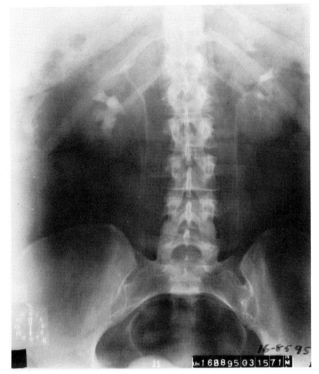

Figure 5–5 (FSB–5). Complete duplication: two ureters pass from the right kidney all the way to the bladder.

may be unilateral or bilateral, incomplete or complete. If the ureters from the two ipsilateral pelves unite to form a common ureter prior to entering the bladder, it is referred to as *incomplete*. When the ureters from the double pelvis enter the bladder separately, the division is referred to as *complete* duplication. Whenever complete duplication occurs, the ureter draining the upper pelvic division crosses the ureter draining the lower pelvic division and inserts into the bladder closer to the bladder neck, so that the upper renal pelvis has the lower ureteral orifice (Figure 5–5, FSB–5; Figure 5–6). This becomes of importance in visualizing the collecting system.

Ectopic ureteral orifices are of clinical importance because when such abnormalities occur they may result in urinary incontinence if beyond the sphincter. They are also prone to obstruction. In the male the ectopic orifice may open into the vesical neck, prostatic urethra, seminal vesicles, vas deferens, or ejaculatory ducts. In the female they may be found in the vesical neck, the urethra, the vagina, the uterus, or the fallopian tubes. In both sexes they may be in the urachus or the rectum. In the

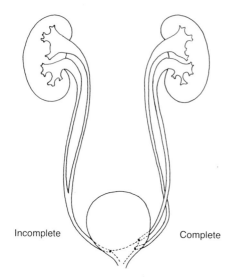

Figure 5-6. Complete and incomplete duplication of ureters. Note crossover in complete duplication.

Incomplete   Complete

case of ureteral duplication in which only one ureteral orifice is ectopic, it is always the one that drains the upper pelvic division.

A *ureterocele* is a cystic dilation of the distal portion of the ureter and is often associated with complete ureteral duplication. Ureteroceles

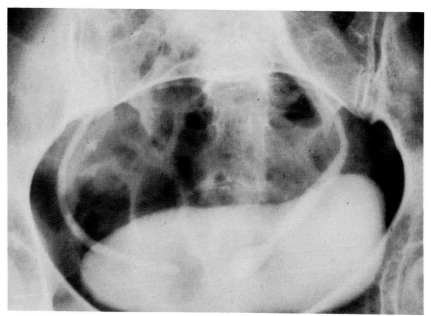

Figure 5-7 (FSB-6). Ureterocele. Note bilateral "cobra head" or "spring onion" image, surrounded by less dense area occupied by bladder and ureteral wall.

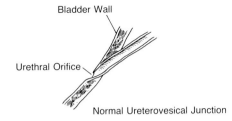

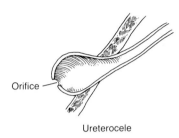

Figure 5-8. Diagram of ureterocele structure.

frequently produce "cobra head" or "spring onion" defects in a bladder
filled with radiopaque contrast material (Figure 5-7, FSB-6). Large ureteroceles may obstruct the bladder neck and even prolapse through the
urethra in females. A ureterocele results from incomplete formation of

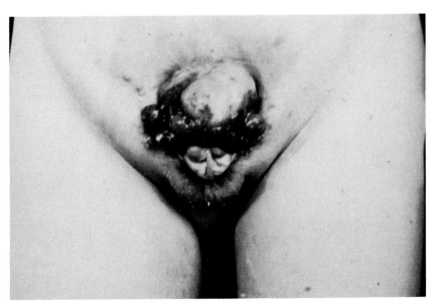

Figure 5-9 (FSB-7). Photograph of patient with exstrophy of bladder. The
dark material is granulation tissue. Note the corpora cavernosa and spongiosum
visible below the dark material. A rudimentary scrotum is also apparent.

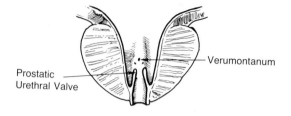

Figure 5–10. Location of prostatic urethral valve.

the opening of the ureter into the bladder. The pinpoint orifice thus formed results in the obstruction and dilation of the ureter (Figure 5–8).

Anomalies of the bladder include a *patent urachus,* which may allow urine to drain from the umbilicus; and *exstrophy of the bladder,* which is characterized by absence of the lower anterior abdominal wall and pubic symphysis separation with eversion of the posterior bladder wall (Figure 5–9, FSB–7). Duplication of the bladder or urethra is rare. *Congenital stricture of the urethra* and *contraction of the bladder neck* are the most common anomalies. These narrowings of the "outflow" tract may be minor in nature and not become clinically evident until adulthood, or it may be so severe that at birth the urinary tract is severely damaged because of the obstruction.

Prostatic urethral valves (Figure 5–10) cause obstruction during urination. This abnormality is usually significant enough to produce a clinical picture of infection or obstruction in early childhood. (These are usually one-way valves; thus the passage of a probe from below may not meet with resistance.) *Hypospadias* (Figure 5–11) is a congenital defect of the anterior urethra in which the urethral opening (meatus) is ventral

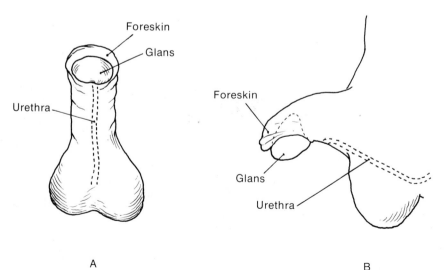

Figure 5–11. Hypospadias.

and proximal to its normal site on the glans penis. This abnormality is of significance because (1) it is frequently associated with meatal stenosis (abnormally small external urethral opening); (2) it is usually associated with chordee (ventral curvature of the penis), Figure 5–11b, which causes a reproductively nonfunctional penis; (3) it may be associated with a meatus located proximally enough on the penile shaft to preclude proper deposit of sperm in the vaginal vault; and (4) cosmetically, the abnormality may be enough to cause psychological problems. Any of these four conditions is reason for surgical correction.

CYSTIC DISEASES

Single (Simple) Cysts (Figure 5–12, FSB–8) are frequent and of little clinical significance. They must, however, be differentiated from primary or metastatic renal tumors, which may also be present clinically as space-occupying nonfunctional renal lesions on the excretory urogram.

Polycystic kidneys (Figure 5–13, FSB–9; Figure 5–14, FSB–10) are important clinically. This abnormality occurs in two distinct forms: one in the infant and one in the adult. In children the disease appears to be genetically transmitted as a Mendelian recessive, whereas in adults it is inherited as a Mendelian dominant with close to 100 per cent penetrance. In children the disease is uniformly fatal with a very short life span. In adults, however, the disease may remain latent for many years, becoming manifest in middle age. The time of appearance of symptoms

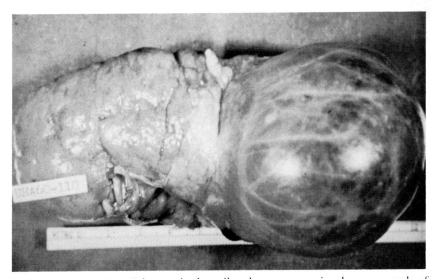

Figure 5–12 (FSB–8). A large, single unilocular cyst occupies the upper pole of this kidney. It is filled with a lucent fluid.

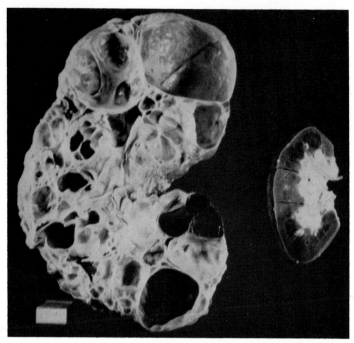

Figure 5–13 (FSB–9). A normal kidney on the right is compared to the large, polycystic one on the left. Note hemorrhage into several of the cysts. The others are filled with a clear fluid. No renal parenchyma is grossly identifiable.

appears to be quite uniform within a family but variable among affected families. The mean age at diagnosis is approximately 50 years, although the range is considerable, extending from 16 years to 85 years.

The most common presenting complaints are hematuria, pain, and a sensation of fullness or pressure in the flank. Polycystic disease predisposes to the development of pyelonephritis and nephrolithiasis (calculi in the collecting system superior to the uretero-pelvic junction). With progressive destruction of the renal parenchyma, hypertension and renal failure develop, usually within 5 to 15 years of the diagnosis. The life span appears to be relatively uniform within one family group.

The lesions of both adult and childhood type are similar and consist of the formation of cysts somewhere along the nephron. In the childhood type the cysts are usually small, although no less numerous than in the adult type, in which the cysts attain a large size, with the kidneys weighing up to 1500 grams. The condition is most often bilateral, although the kidneys may not be equally large. Within one kidney the cysts vary from microscopic to several centimeters in diameter. They usually communicate with the nephron, which retains some function until obstruction and increased pressure intervene. Progressive dilation of the cysts, with compression of the interstitium and surrounding nephrons, is the presumed mechanism for progressive interstitial fibrosis. Compression and stasis also predispose to infection, thus increasing the fibrosis. Commonly associated with polycystic kidneys are cysts of the liver and berry aneurysms of the circle of Willis. The cause of death in these patients is most often terminal renal failure, although hypertensive heart disease and rupture of intracerebral aneurysms may occur.

The diagnosis of polycystic renal disease may be suspected from a positive family history, patient awareness of increasing abdominal fullness, or the presence of large, palpable kidneys. The diagnosis is confirmed by an excretory urogram (IVP, see p. 240) in which kidneys are seen to be diffusely enlarged, and the calyces assume an elongated thin (stretched) appearance (Figure 5–14, FSB–10). It is important to note that liver disease (cysts with fibrosis) is a common accompaniment of the childhood form and may lead to liver failure before renal failure.

There is no definitive treatment of polycystic renal disease. Surgical drainage of the cysts does not improve function and is complicated by the development of infection. Instrumentation is to be avoided if possible.

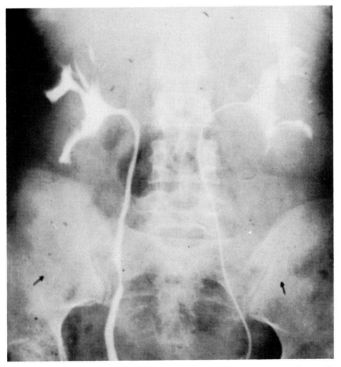

Figure 5–14 (FSB–10). Polycystic kidneys. Both kidneys are enlarged, and the calyces are spread out and flattened by multiple cysts.

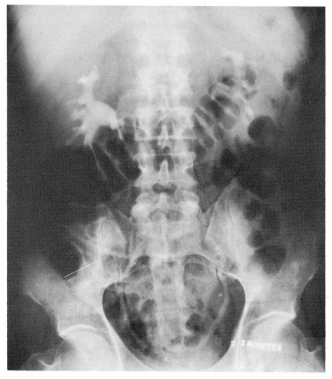

Figure 5–15 (FSB–11). Sponge kidney. Note filling of dilated collecting ducts (beyond normal calyces) with contrast medium.

Medullary cysts are seen in two diseases, one essentially benign and the other with a very poor prognosis. *Medullary sponge kidney* (renal tubular ectasia, non-uremic medullary cystic disease) is characterized by cystic dilation of the papillary collecting ducts. Radiographic examination shows filling of the dilated ducts and apparent stasis of the contrast material (Figure 5–15, FSB–11). The condition is entirely benign and the significance of recognizing medullary sponge kidney is the tendency to form stones in the dilated ducts with resultant hematuria, obstruction, and infection.

The serious form, *medullary cystic disease,* differs from polycystic disease in that most of the cysts are confined to the medulla. Medullary cystic disease is variably transmitted. The patients present with a history of polyuria and refractory, normochromic anemia. They are found to have salt wasting and interstitial nephritis with progressive renal failure.

RENAL PARENCHYMAL DISEASES, GENERAL

Excluding its production of specific hormones, the major task performed by the kidney is ultrafiltration of the plasma, selective reabsorption of parts of the filtrate, and secretion of various substances into the tubular lumina. All of these processes are regulated within rather narrow limits, and aberrations are reflected by a change in the quality or quantity of the end product—urine. Recognition of renal disease depends on observable changes in the urine. The type of change seen reflects the site and severity of the change induced in each area. For instance, when protein is present in excessive quantities in the urine, an abnormality in that segment of the nephron which normally excludes protein from the filtrate, the glomerulus, should be immediately suspected. As a matter of fact, the presence of proteinuria is the best clinical indicator of the presence of glomerular disease. This same general concept can be applied to each anatomic and functional unit. In order that some sense may be made from the multiple histopathological, functional, and clinical presentations of renal disease, the basic responses to injury should be considered and applied to each segment of the kidney. The consequences of the stimulus can then be predicted.

The following sections are designed to aid in the development of an understanding of the responses of the kidney to diverse stimuli in terms of the basic pathologic processes. Rather than provide a catalog of exotic diseases with mystic causes and uncertain prognosis, it is the intent to provide an organizational framework for placing future observations and data in useful perspective.

Glomerular Disease

A clear understanding of glomerular disease rests on a consideration of the normal glomerular structure and the basic pathologic changes which are possible. The glomerulus consists of cells and extracellular material (ECM); the possible cellular changes are: (1) an increase in number *(hyperplasia)*; (2) a decrease in number *(atrophy)*; (3) *necrosis*; and (4) *exudation* (infiltration by neutrophils). The possible extracellular changes are: (1) an increase in amount of ECM *(sclerosis* or *scarring)*; and (2) accumulation of foreign protein *(deposits)*. Any or all of these processes may coexist in one patient. Their extent and severity correlate with immediate function and long-term prognosis. Tables 5–1 and 5–2 summarize the changes and their characteristics.

It is important to note that the cellular and extracellular processes noted above may involve *all of every* glomerulus (diffuse change), *all of a few* glomeruli (focal change), or *part of a few* glomeruli (local change). Both the focal and local changes have been referred to as *focal* in previous descriptions.

Table 5-1.   Cellular Changes.

PROCESS	Neutrophils	Endothelial	Mesangial	Epithelial	ABNORMALITY
	CELL TYPE				
Hyperplasia		X	X		diffuse hypercellularity (proliferation), Figure 5-16a, FSB-12
"				X	crescent (if it involves the whole glomerulus), Figure 5-16b, FSB-13
"				X	synechia (if it involves only part of the glomerulus), Figure 5-16c, FSB-14
"	X				exudation (may accompany any of the above), Figure 5-16d, FSB-15
Decrease or atrophy		X	X	X	This change may be seen in any long-standing glomerular disease which results in sclerosis (scarring). The end-stage of this process is, of course, obsolescence.
Necrosis		X	X	X	Especially common in crescents.

If the above concepts are not clear, stop and start again at the beginning, because a clear understanding of the following discussion is predicated on assimilation of this information.

Definition of Glomerulonephritis

The term "glomerulonephritis" literally means "inflammation of the glomeruli and tubules (the nephron)." Through common usage, however, *any change presumed primarily to affect the glomeruli,* even sclerosis (scarring), *is called "glomerulonephritis."* Thus, the glomerular lesion, characterized by uniform, glomerular basement membrane thickening and glomerular *hypocellularity,* is called "membranous glomerulonephritis." While incorrect, such uses of the term "glomerulonephritis" are too deeply ingrained in medical literature to be easily discarded. The simplest way to think of glomerulonephritis is that it is a nonspecific inflammatory response of the kidney thought primarily to affect the glomeruli. Ordinarily, the glomeruli are the most conspicuously involved; however, the tubules and interstitium are also affected. Characteristically, the major urinary findings of a glomerular change are hematuria and proteinuria, including red blood cell casts. The RBC cast is pathognomonic of glomerular disease, so much so in fact that it is

Text continued on page 157.

Table 5-2. Extracellular Material Changes.

PROCESS	LOCATION		CHANGE
	GBM	Mesangial Matrix	
Increase	X		membranous change, Figure 5-17a,b (FSB-16, FSB-17)
Increase	X	X	glomerulosclerosis (Note: When the glomerular basement membrane thickens in a uniform manner, the mesangial matrix is usually also increased.) This is the change associated with diabetes mellitus.

PROCESS	LOCATION				CHANGE
Deposits	Subepithelial	Intramembranous	Subendothelial	Mesangial	
Diffuse (regular)	X				present in so-called "membranous glomerulonephritis," Figure 5-18 (FSB-18
Diffuse (irregular or granular)	X				present in most straightforward post-infectious antigen-antibody nephritides, Figure 5-17d,e (FSB-19, FSB-20)
				X	as the lesion heals, the deposits are found primarily in the mesangial regions
Focal			X	X	forms "wire loop" lesion typical of systemic lupus erythematosus (SLE) (also present in other diseases, Figure 5-17f,g (FSB-21, FSB-22)
		X		X	deposits may be within or on the endothelial aspect in membranoproliferative or mesangiocapillary disease

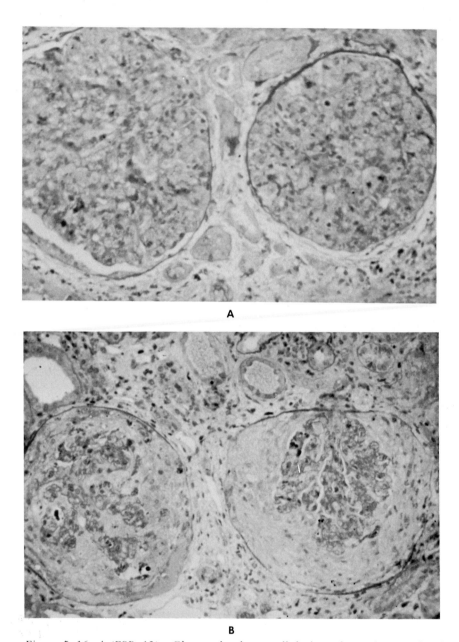

Figure 5–16. A (FSB–12), Glomerular hypercellularity: photomicrograph of two glomeruli with diffuse increase in the number of intraglomerular cells. *B (FSB–13)*, Epithelial crescent: photograph of a glomerulus with proliferation of epithelial cells filling Bowman's space and compressing glomerular capillaries.

Figure 5–16 *continued on opposite page.*

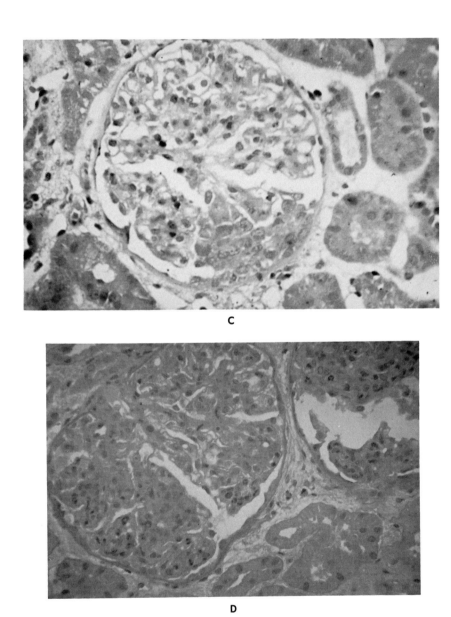

Figure 5-16. C *(FSB-14)*, Synechia: epithelial cell proliferation compromises only a small part of Bowman's space. D *(FSB-15)*, Exudation: glomerulus with diffuse intraglomerular proliferation and many polymorphonuclear leukocytes.

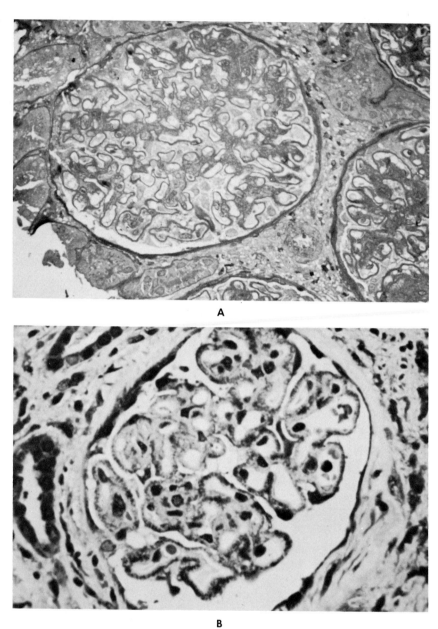

A

B

Figure 5–17. A (FSB–16), Diffuse GBM thickening: two glomeruli with a diffuse, uniform increase in the thickness of the glomerular basement membranes. Also note that the mesangial regions are prominent. *B (FSB–17),* Trichrome stain of a glomerulus with diffuse basement membrane thickening and uniform, diffuse distribution of subepithelial deposits.

Figure 5–17 *continued on opposite page.*

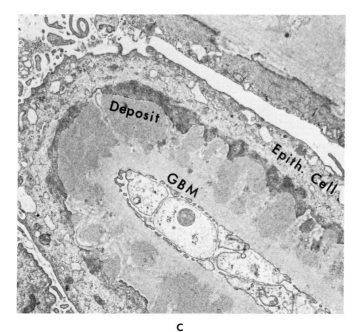

C

D

Figure 5–17. C (FSB–18), Electron micrograph of the same biopsy with diffuse regular subepithelial deposits. Note fusion of the epithelial foot processes. The Bowman's membrane at the side is also thickened. *D (FSB–19),* Trichrome stain of a glomerulus from a patient with irregular subepithelial deposits scattered over multiple capillary loops. The patient had post-streptococcal glomerulonephritis.

Figure 5–17 *continued on following page.*

156 DISEASES OF THE URINARY TRACT

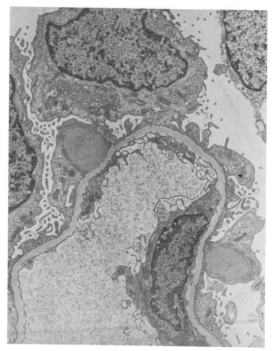

E

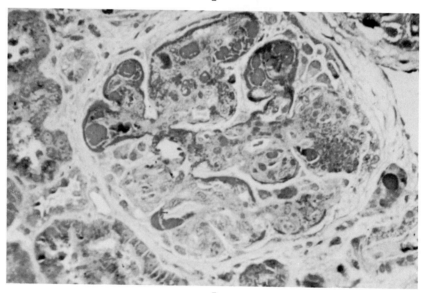

F

Figure 5–17. E (FSB–20), Electron micrograph demonstrating normal-appearing glomerular basement membrane with irregular subepithelial deposits in a patient with post-streptococcal glomerulonephritis. *F (FSB–21),* Trichrome stain of a glomerulus with subendothelial deposits; note the many large, dark deposits scattered throughout the glomerulus in subendothelial locations.

Figure 5–17 *continued on opposite page.*

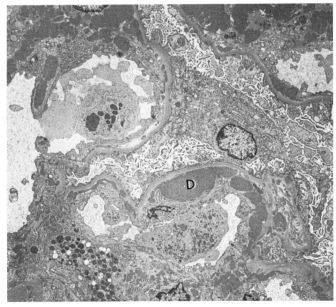

G

Figure 5-17. G *(FSB-22),* Electron micrograph from same patient as F. Note the large subendothelial deposits (D) present in several capillary loops. There is focal fusion of epithelial foot processes as well.

referred to as "glomerular bleeding." As expected, a primarily sclerosing process has less hematuria and RBC casts than an active inflammatory process.

Classification of Glomerulonephritis

The classification of glomerulonephritides is currently undergoing a substantial change. However, the terms *acute, subacute, latent,* and *chronic* glomerulonephritis are still used by many people. For these reasons, it is imperative to have a clear understanding of what is meant by each term.

The following historical sketch will illustrate how the current nomenclature of renal disease was derived. Morgagni, in the 18th century, was the first physician systematically to study and record the relationships between structure and function. The father of the investigation of renal disease was Richard Bright. He used very simple methods to detect renal disease (boiling urine in a pewter spoon over a tallow candle and then adding a drop of vinegar to check for a coagulum—protein). Others had noted a similar change in urine, but Bright was the first to carefully follow the patients to the end stages of renal disease. He con-

Table 5-3. Classifications According to Volhard and Fahr.

CATEGORY	CLINICAL FINDINGS		PROGNOSIS	LAB. FINDINGS	ANATOMIC FINDINGS	
	Onset	*Physical Findings*			*Gross*	*Histologic*
Acute	rapid	edema, mild hyper-tension	excellent	proteinuria, RBC, RBC casts	enlarged kidneys	diffusely hypercellular; enlarged, bloodless glomeruli containing many neutrophils (proliferation & exudation)
Subacute	insidious	edema, mild hyper-tension	rapid pro-gression to renal failure	proteinuria, RBC, RBC casts (the patient may have an elevated creatinine when first seen)	enlarged kidneys	glomerular hypercellularity (primarily epithelial cells—*crescents*)
Chronic	insidious	hypertension, edema, polyuria	slow pro-gression to renal failure	proteinuria, RBC's, casts (granular & occasional RBC)	small & scarred	end-stage; that is, scarring has so affected the architecture that the original process is not discernible

vincingly demonstrated that those with constant "albuminous urine" had diseased kidneys. The term *Bright's disease* was then coined and was used to refer to any kidney malady associated with proteinuria. In the period from 1827 to 1914 a seemingly endless variety of clinical conditions thought to be due to malfunction of the kidney was recognized. Many showed protein in the urine. The problem was that some patients did well, in spite of marked proteinuria, and some died from rapidly advancing renal failure. Physicians were in a quandary concerning how to deal conceptually with this problem. In 1914, Volhard and Fahr took advantage of the advances in medicine since Bright's time, carefully followed patients with renal diseases, and noted that they could be divided into a limited number of categories depending on *clinical presentation*. They also found that the gross and histologic *anatomic findings* at autopsy could be classified according to a scheme based on the primary pathologic processes. The categories in Table 5–3 were described.

These observations formed the foundations of their classification of renal disease. It is this classification under which we labor today. The first category, characterized by a rapid onset of illness with a favorable prognosis, was called *acute* glomerulonephritis. Those with a similar onset but whose disease, rather than resolving, pursued a stormy downhill course to renal failure, were placed in the category of *subacute* (non-healing) glomerulonephritis. Finally, when the initial diagnosis depended on the chance finding of proteinuria and the clinical course to renal failure was measured in decades, the process was called *chronic* glomerulonephritis. The designations acute, subacute, and chronic suggest a temporal sequence of disease. Since renal disease rarely, if ever, evolves from acute to subacute and then chronic, the terms are misleading.

This classification does not suffice for modern medicine. With the advent of percutaneous biopsy, we now recognize that the number of diseases associated with cellular proliferation in the glomeruli is *staggering*—to call them all "acute glomerulonephritis" obscures rather than aids in establishing the proper diagnosis, prognosis, and treatment plan. The same may be said for changes in the quantity of extracellular material. A more meaningful method of describing renal disease (making a diagnosis) is to state the extent of one's knowledge of the disease, utilizing all of the parameters available. Note how much more information is conveyed by the diagnosis "proliferative and exudative glomerulonephritis following streptococcal pharyngitis," rather than the simple appelation "acute glomerulonephritis." The former description indicates the etiology and pathologic processes, and allows one to arrive at the correct prognosis and therapy.

A few generalizations about glomerulonephritis may be made. Most of the histologic reactions considered characteristic of glomerulonephritis are commonly thought to involve only the glomeruli. In fact, the glomeruli are but one part of a large renal capillary system. Only very recently have we appreciated that many (if not all) capillary beds exhibit responses to injury similar to those seen in glomeruli. Therefore, if a diffuse reaction of great severity occurs in the glomerular capillary bed, interstitial and tubular disease would be expected as well. This is, in fact, the observed association. Similarly, "capillaritis" may be manifest in other capillary beds (muscles, resulting in myalgia; central nervous system, resulting in seizures; etc.).

It would be logical to assume that the kidney would primarily react to stimuli delivered by the circulatory system, since this is its major contact with the "outside world." Those substances, other than chemical toxins (poisons), about which we know the most are humoral, immunologic reactions. There are at least two varieties of immunologic injury. One is due to *antigen-antibody (Ag-Ab) complexes* which become lodged in the glomeruli by virtue of their filtration function. Second, there are *anti-kidney* antibodies directed against a specific part of the kidney; those directed against the glomerular basement membrane (anti-GBM) have been most extensively studied. Antigen-antibody complexes produce an evanescent lesion with little residual effect unless (1) there is a continued source of antigen, in which case the process is never resolved, or (2) the first insult was so severe as to result in massive damage. By way of contrast, most renal diseases associated with anti-GBM antibody result in severe, permanent renal injury. Fortunately, this is an uncommon form of renal disease, whereas antigen-antibody complex nephritis is very common.

The source of antigens which may be associated with antigen-antibody nephritis includes bacteria, viruses, plasmodia (malaria), and drugs (penicillin). In short, any antigen to which circulating antibody may be formed can evoke this reaction. Included in this category is a group of diseases in which the antigen is thought to be *autogenous,* that is, some antigen is normally present in the body. This group comprises the *auto-immune* or *collagen-vascular* diseases. Since the source of antigen is continuously present, this form of nephritis results in significant and frequently progressive renal damage.

A current immunology text will give complete details of the mechanism of injury following deposition of Ag-Ab complexes or attachment of antibody to GBM. It is important to recognize that complement is fixed to antigen-antibody complexes and a series of reactions ensues which leads to chemotaxis of neutrophils and release of proteases, vasoactive amines, and other substances. Capillary permeability increases and proteins and cells leak outside of their vascular confines. An increase in permeability in the glomerular capillaries results in protein and red blood cells in the tubules (and eventually in the urine, where they are recognized as proteinuria, hematuria, and RBC casts). In peritubular capillaries an increase in capillary permeability results in interstitial edema and a leukocytic infiltrate. Neutrophils may accentuate tissue destruction by release of hydrolytic enzymes from their many lysosomes. Since the formation of soluble antigen-antibody complexes is an evanescent affair in most infectious diseases, the complexes are quickly phagocytized and the injury resolves. If the antigen persists, as in chronic infection, the injury is cumulative and results in distortion of the tissue by scarring and actual loss of nephrons.

It is conceivable that the severe lesions seen in the presence of anti-GBM antibody result from the fact that in order to get rid of the Ag-Ab complex, the GBM must also be removed and the glomerulus becomes totally disrupted and nonfunctional.

Proliferative Glomerulonephritis

The glomerulonephritis of immunologic origin belongs to the histological class of proliferative glomerulonephritis, often called acute GN in the older nomenclature because of sudden onset and the associated cellular proliferation and exudation. There are many examples of renal disease which share these histologic features but do *not* appear to be immunologically mediated.

Post-streptococcal Glomerulonephritis: An example of an Evanescent Ag-Ab Complex Nephritis. The most common form of Ag-Ab glomerulonephritis in children is that seen following infections with β-hemolytic streptococci. Type 12 is the most frequently implicated strain, but others have been reported in various epidemics. The pharynx is often quoted as the usual site of infection, although the skin is frequently involved in cases in the southern part of the U.S.A.

The relationship between streptococcal infections and proliferative glomerulonephritis is established, but the exact pathogenesis of the disease is far from clear. It is clear that there is no direct involvement of the kidney by intact organisms. A direct effect by a bacterial product is also not likely, since the bacterial infection has cleared before a renal lesion becomes manifest.

The most likely possibility is that the nephritis is due to trapping of antigen-antibody complexes in the kidney. The deposition of the complexes on the glomerular basement membrane is followed by fixation of complement and subsequent damage by the proteases liberated in the complement reaction, as well as by neutrophils attracted by the liberated chemotactic factors. As is true of most antigen-antibody complex nephritides where the antigen appears only transiently, the injury is evanescent and heals rapidly.

The appearance of oliguria or anuria is related to the severity of the interstitial and tubular changes. Interstitial edema interferes with cortical perfusion by compressing peritubular capillaries, and it also interferes with diffusion of reabsorbed material from proximal tubular epithelial cells into the surrounding capillaries by increasing the distance between the capillary lumen and tubular cell. This aspect of the nephritis is ordinarily mild and, therefore, oliguria is often not clinically apparent.

There are four phases in the acute disease: (1) infection, (2) latent, (3) nephritis, and (4) healing. The *acute infection* may be so mild as to pass unnoticed by the patient. This is an important phase, however, since synthesis of antibodies to bacterial antigens begins here. After a *latent period* of 10 to 14 days the *nephritic* period begins. This corresponds to the time when serum antistreptococcal antibody reaches high enough titers to form soluble Ag-Ab complexes which localize in capillary beds, especially those of the kidney. The clinical result is edema, malaise, mild and usually transient hypertension, and an "active" urinary sediment containing red blood cells, red blood cell casts, and protein. The urine assumes a "smoky" or reddish color because of the abnormal constituents and may be decreased in volume. Anuria is uncommon. Oliguria is not infrequent but only roughly correlates with the severity of the glomerular disease. After a short period of oliguria, diuresis ensues. The number of formed elements in the urine (cells and casts) diminishes rapidly. Mild proteinuria and hematuria may persist for considerably longer periods or reappear during minor illnesses for many months.

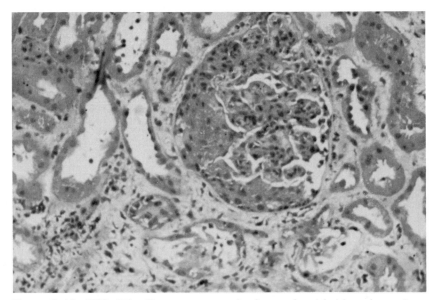

Figure 5-18 (FSB-23). Post-streptococcal glomerulonephritis: photomicrograph demonstrating proliferative and exudative changes within glomerular tufts. There is also epithelial cell hyperplasia. Note the edema of the surrounding interstitial tissue.

The presence of prolonged proteinuria signals persistent renal disease. During the acute phase of the illness, there may be a modestly elevated BUN (blood urea nitrogen), mild anemia, and elevated serum cholesterol (especially in children). Streptolysin O, streptococcal hyaluronidase, and streptokinase antibody titers rise rapidly and remain elevated for a considerable period of time. If all three antibodies are measured, over 95 percent of patients with recent streptococcal infections can be identified, while the figure drops to 75 percent if only anti-streptolysin-O titers are determined. Since the prognosis of post-streptococcal glomerulonephritis is benign compared to other diseases associated with glomerulonephritis in this age group, this diagnosis is crucial.

Histologically, post-streptococcal glomerulonephritis is a diffuse, inflammatory reaction of the glomeruli with variable tubular and interstitial involvement (Figure 5-18, FSB-23; Figure 5-19, FSB-24; Figure 5-20, FSB-25). There is prominent cellular proliferation and hyperplasia. Neutrophils, macrophages, and eosinophils may also be present in the exudative form. Large, irregular subepithelial deposits, composed of IgG and complement, are present on the glomerular basement membranes.

The prognosis in post-streptococcal glomerulonephritis in children appears to be entirely benign. Even when there are prolonged periods of oliguria or anuria associated with the acute event, persistent proteinuria or renal failure rarely occurs. The same thing may be true in adults, although the evidence is not as clear in this age group.

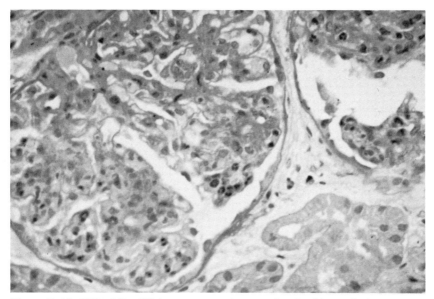

Figure 5-19 (FSB-24). Higher power micrograph of subject of Figure 5-18. Note the presence of neutrophils within the capillary lumen.

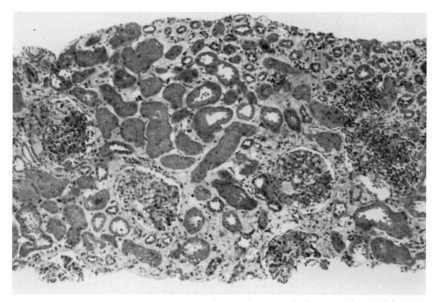

Figure 5-20 (FSB-25). Low-power photomicrograph from patient with post-streptococcal glomerulonephritis. Note the interstitial edema and infiltrate separating tubules.

Systemic Lupus Erythematosus (SLE) Nephritis: An Ag-Ab Complex Disease In Which There Is Persistence Of Antigen. The presence of antinuclear antibodies and low complement levels in the serum of patients with active SLE suggests that patients are producing antibodies to their own tissues. Even if this proves to be of importance in the pathogenesis of the disease, the nature of the initiating event is unclear. SLE is a multi-system disease which produces major morphologic alterations both of the connective tissue which separates and supports cells and of the small blood vessels. Hence it is one of the "collagen-vascular" diseases. It affects young females more often than males (10/1) and is characterized by fever, photosensitive skin rashes, arthritis, anemia, leukopenia, lymphadenopathy, pleuritis, pericarditis, and neurologic and renal involvement. The characteristic features of SLE are involvement of many different tissues and wide variation in clinical expression. The first form to be recognized was a rapidly advancing, usually fatal, systemic illness characterized by all of the abnormalities mentioned above. At the other end of the spectrum lies an indolent, remitting disease characterized by arthralgia, myalgia, and malaise. Degrees of severity between these extremes are common. Not only is the disease characterized by enormous variability in its clinical forms, but the extent and severity of involvement of different organ systems may change during the illness. Even when severe manifestations of the disease are present, they *may* spontaneously disappear, making evaluation of therapy difficult.

Renal involvement may occur early in the disease and is found in about 50 percent of patients at the time of initial diagnosis. There is no correlation between the severity of SLE and the presence or absence of renal disease. It is rare, however, for those initially without renal disease to develop involvement later on. Renal disease sufficient to produce azotemia is an ominous sign and the cause of death in about 30 percent of patients so affected. When glomerular renal disease is present, it falls into one of the following groups: (1) diffuse proliferation (lupus GN) (Figure 5–21, FSB–26); (2) focal proliferation (Figure 5–22, FSB–27); or (3) sclerosis (membranous GN) (Figure 5–23, FSB–28). Although the overlap between clinical presentation and pathological categorization is great, it does appear that the presence of active glomerular inflammation and damage correlate closely with activity of SLE in other systems. The following generalizations can be made: (1) those with diffuse proliferation usually follow a rapidly progressive deterioration with eventual renal failure; (2) those with focal proliferation may have a very active urinary sediment, but the lesion seldom progresses; (3) those with sclerosis follow a course similar to other patients with membranous glomerulonephritis; (4) those without significant proteinuria or urinary sediment abnormalities most often have no renal disease and seldom develop this

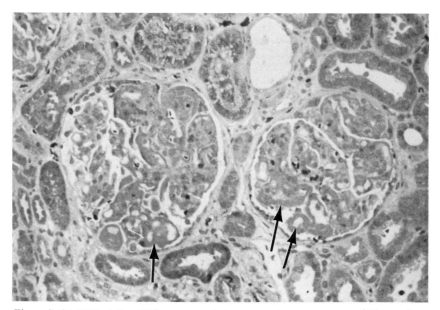

Figure 5–21 (FSB–26). Diffuse systemic lupus erythematosus: renal biopsy from patient, showing diffuse proliferation of intraglomerular cells involving all glomeruli with multiple deposits (arrows). Note the interstitial edema and mononuclear infiltrate.

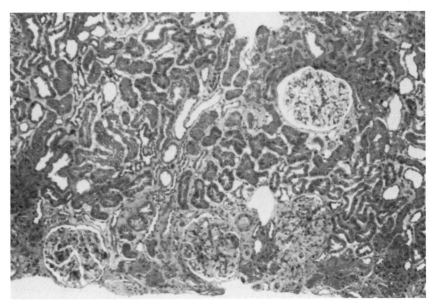

Figure 5-22 (FSB-27). Focal systemic lupus erythematosus: low-power photomicrograph demonstrating irregular distribution of changes between glomeruli. One is normal and others show varying changes.

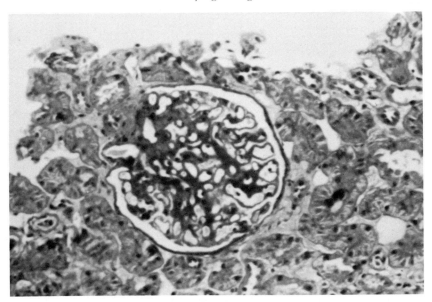

Figure 5-23 (FSB-28). Membranous lesion in systemic lupus erythematosus: glomerulus with diffuse uniform thickening of glomerular basement membranes. Note that in this case the glomeruli are not hypercellular; rather, they appear hypocellular.

complication; and (5) there is little tendency for either focal proliferation or sclerosis to progress to diffuse proliferation.

The morphologic characteristics reflect the general severity of the
disease. Diffuse glomerulonephritis in SLE is characterized by large, pale
kidneys similar to those with severe or rapidly progressive GN. Microscopically, there may be proliferation of all glomerular cell types with
crescents, synechiae, and other features characteristic of flagrant disease. However, the changes between glomeruli are often irregular.
There is frequently necrosis within tufts, and characteristically there are
large focal subendothelial deposits (the so-called wire loop lesions of
SLE) (Figure 5–17g; Figure 5–24, FSB–29). The deposits contain IgG,
IgM, and complement (Figure 5–25, FSB–30). Viral-like inclusions have
been described in the endothelial cells. In areas of necrosis, collections
of amorphous nuclear material (hematoxylin bodies) may be seen. The
interstitium commonly contains large numbers of plasma cells and
lymphocytes. The presence of the former is taken by some as evidence
of an active disease. Changes in large vessels are infrequent and when
present may be related to hypertension.

**Rapidly Progressive Glomerulonephritis (RPGN): In Part an
Anti-GBM Nephritis.** This is a form of GN which pursues a rapid (6 to
18 months) course ending in renal failure. Post-streptococcal GN very
infrequently follows this course. The majority of patients with rapidly
progressive GN have no previous history or laboratory data suggesting a

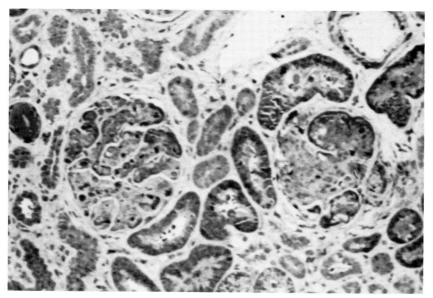

Figure 5–24 (FSB–29). Trichrome stain of diffuse systemic lupus erythematosus, showing multiple subendothelial deposits.

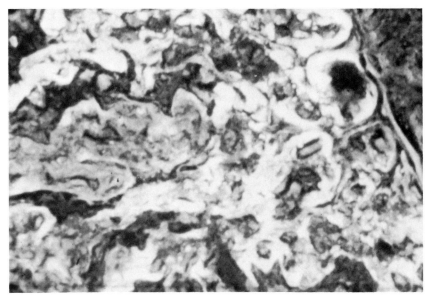

Figure 5–25 (FSB–30). Systemic lupus erythematosus: fluorescence micrograph of a glomerulus stain with anti-gamma G, demonstrating multiple subendothelial deposits as well as many deposits within mesangial regions.

preceding streptococcal infection. The clinical course is that of increasing azotemia and a falling GFR. Hypertension is frequently present, especially if sodium intake is not restricted. The urine contains protein, RBC's, and casts of all types. Although RBC, renal tubular, and granular are most frequent, WBC, waxy, fatty, and broad casts are also seen. The finding of this wide spectrum of casts (a telescopic urine sediment) is highly suggestive of RPGN. Spontaneous recovery appears to be rare.

Grossly, the kidneys are large, pale, and edematous. The glomeruli are diffusely affected. The most striking change is that of marked parietal glomerular epithelial cell proliferation (Figure 5–26, FSB–31) which reduces or obliterates Bowman's space, forming a *crescent.* The crescents, depending on the duration of the illness, may be quite dense, with the spaces between cells being filled with a collagen or basement membrane-like material. Deposits or specific features have not been seen by electron microscopy. In approximately ⅓ of the cases fluorescence microscopy reveals linear deposits of IgG on the GBM's (Figure 5–27, FSB–32). Within the tuft there may be cellular proliferation similar to that seen in post-streptococcal GN, but it is not usually as florid or regular. Necrosis and sclerosis are common.

Tubular changes are often florid and consist of necrosis and proliferation of epithelial cells. The interstitium is edematous and infiltrated with inflammatory cells. Vascular changes are not prominent until

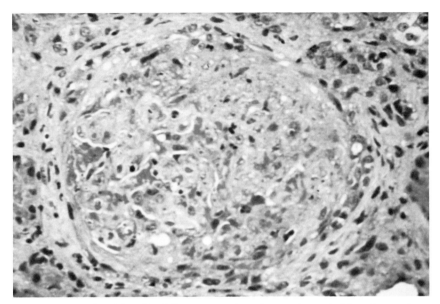

Figure 5-26 (FSB-31). Rapidly progressive glomerulonephritis: photomicrograph of a glomerulus in which it is difficult to identify any normal landmarks because of marked proliferation of cells outside the glomerular tuft. The dark streaks within Bowman's capsule are collections of fibrin and other serum proteins. Glomerular basement membranes are not identifiable.

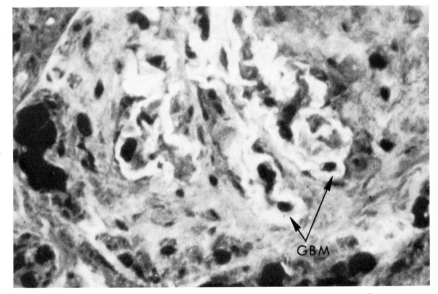

Figure 5-27 (FSB-32). Rapidly progressive glomerulonephritis: fluorescence micrograph with staining by anti-gamma G. Note the linear staining of the glomerular basement membranes (arrows). The outlines of Bowman's capsule are seen faintly in the periphery, as are a number of cells within Bowman's space.

hypertension is seen, at which time the interlobular arteries are most prominently affected (see p. 184).

The etiology of this lesion is puzzling. The majority of patients have no clinical, bacteriologic, or serologic evidence of bacterial or viral infection. In some cases it has been shown that anti-GBM antibody is fixed to the glomeruli. The antibody can be found in the serum of these patients if the kidneys are removed. The majority of patients do not have a circulating antibody to GBM in their serum.

A similar renal lesion may be associated with other systemic illnesses such as SLE and the microangiopathic form of periarteritis nodosa. In these instances there are usually other means to establish the correct diagnosis. RPGN is, therefore, a clinico-pathologic description rather than an etiologic diagnosis.

Other Forms of Proliferative Glomerulonephritis. Many forms of proliferative GN have been described which do not appear to be associated with a humoral immunologic response. Some are a significant part of well-defined clinical syndromes like Henoch-Schönlein purpura, however, and deserve mention from that standpoint.

Henoch-Schönlein purpura is a disease, primarily of children, characterized by the abrupt onset of lower extremity rash, abdominal pain, joint pain and, less commonly, GI bleeding. The renal lesion presents primarily as a focal proliferative and exudative glomerular lesion. In the absence of the characteristic clinical manifestations of the disease, the "nephritis" may be extremely difficult to differentiate from any other type of focal glomerular change. Like the other manifestations of the disease, the nephritis seems to disappear in children without residual damage. Permanent renal damage has been reported in adults.

A completely benign form of *focal glomerular cell proliferation* has recently been recognized in adults. This condition is most often detected upon examination of a routinely obtained urine sample which is found to contain red blood cells, protein, and RBC casts. The sediment abnormalities may disappear, only to reappear after minor illnesses. The significance of this condition is that the overwhelming majority of these patients do well over a long period of time, in contrast to those with many other renal diseases showing similar urinary sediment changes. The diagnosis must be confirmed by renal biopsy. The anatomic picture is similar to that described in Henoch-Schönlein purpura and consists of a localized proliferation of cells within the glomerular tuft, affecting only a small number of glomeruli (a focal pattern).

Renal Diseases Associated with Increased ECM (Chronic or Sclerosing GN's)

Many of the previously discussed types of GN represent examples of diseases with a dramatic, often explosive onset and an equally vivid outcome. However, the majority of patients with renal disease are discovered as the result of an abnormal urinalysis. Their disease has a prolonged course and only very slowly, if at all, progresses to renal failure. Any one patient may have multiple episodes of acute renal inflammatory disease superimposed on his chronic disease, but the general course of the GN appears to remain the same within broad limits. Patients with this clinical picture and who have some evidence of decreased renal function (elevated creatinine or BUN) are said to have chronic GN.

These forms of GN are anatomically characterized by slowly increasing sclerosis of the renal parenchyma. In the presence of hematuria, RBC casts in the urinary sediment, and some degree of proteinuria, a diagnosis of GN is made. Although clinical knowledge of the duration of the disease is useful, the diagnosis of sclerosing GN, short of a renal biopsy, cannot be made unless an impairment of renal function is present.

Chronic GN is most frequently diagnosed between ages 20 and 40, but it is commonly found above and below these limits. There appears to be no sex difference in most large series. Frequently, the presence of renal disease is suspected by the observation of proteinuria on a routine checkup, an episode of unexplained edema, or the appearance of hypertension. The detection of protein in the urine gives no clue to the type or extent of renal involvement. In most studies of patients with proteinuria, there has been noted extreme variability (2 to 30 years) in the length of time a patient remained in this stage of the illness before renal function ceased. It is quite clear, however, that many patients with proteinuria never become uremic.

Chronic or sclerosing GN represents the *final common pathway* of a number of diseases. The causes of the original lesion may be quite diverse and are often impossible to determine. In some cases the initial insult might have been post-streptococcal GN, but in the majority of patients no clear-cut history of acute nephritis is obtained.

The histology of chronic GN will vary, but there are two broad, fairly distinct histologic categories: a proliferative form and a membranous form. The latter is associated with uniformly and diffusely thickened GBM's. The clinical presentation also varies: significant proteinuria and even the nephrotic syndrome may be seen in association with the membranous form early in the course of the disease. In the proliferative variety heavy proteinuria is not common until later in the disease, and usually at a time when renal failure is imminent.

The proliferative form of CGN is characterized grossly by small kidneys (20 to 30 per cent of normal) (Figure 5–28, FSB–33) with finely pitted cortical surfaces, especially in those patients with proliferative and sclerosing GN. The cortex is thinned and fibrotic. No changes are seen in the medulla or pelvis. Histologically there is a background of glomerular hypercellularity still visible in the sclerotic kidney (Figure

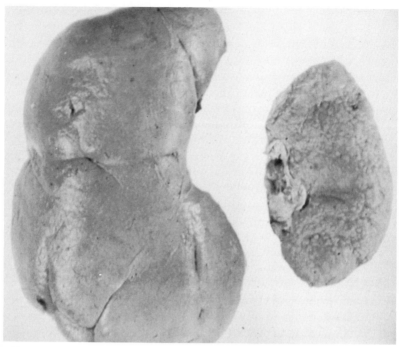

Figure 5-28 (FSB-33). End-stage renal disease: gross photograph of a small, scarred, granular kidney from a patient with chronic glomerulonephritis, compared to a normal kidney.

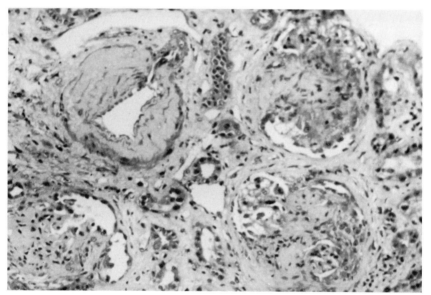

Figure 5-29 (FSB-34). Chronic glomerulonephritis: photomicrograph of three glomeruli, showing varying degrees of sclerosis. Note that the interstitium is also scarred, and the adjacent vessel has duplication of the internal elastic lamellae.

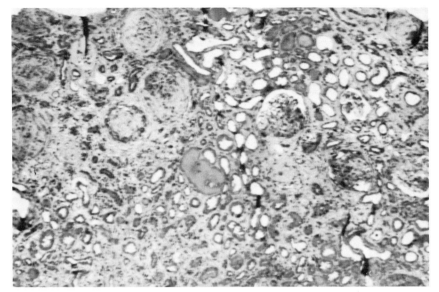

Figure 5–30 (FSB–35). Advanced proliferative glomerulonephritis: low-power photomicrograph emphasizing the irregularity of involvement of glomeruli. Some are completely obsolescent, and an occasional one is relatively normal.

5–29, FSB–34). Glomerular changes secondary to hypertension are difficult to distinguish from those due to the primary disease and, indeed, it may be impossible to separate the two. Most glomeruli are involved and often to a variable extent (Figure 5–30, FSB–35). Many obsolescent glomeruli are seen. Synechiae, crescents, and partial sclerosis of the glomeruli are frequent findings. The basement membrane of the glomerulus is focally, but not uniformly, thickened. When there is shrinkage and partial sclerosis of the tuft producing a lobular pattern, the disease is called chronic lobular GN. Tubular atrophy is always present. The extent of this change is inversely related to kidney size and directly related to the severity of the glomerular disease. The vascular changes are those of hypertension and will be discussed in a later section.

A variant with both sclerosis and proliferation has recently been described. Immunoglobulin deposits and mesangial proliferation characterize this morphologic pattern, which has been labeled mesangiocapillary GN (Figure 5–31, FSB–36) (see below).

The kidneys are often large or normal sized in those with the membranous form of CGN. The cortex is often normal in width in the latter but, like those with proliferative and sclerosing GN, the parenchyma is firm and "gritty" because of the extensive sclerosis.

The *membranous form of CGN* is characterized histologically by a uniform diffuse thickening of the glomerular basement membranes (Figure

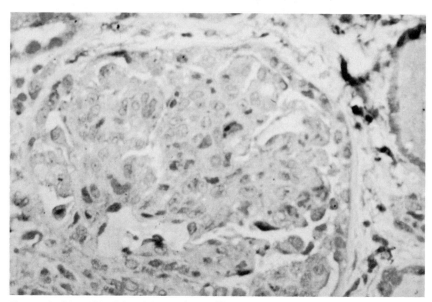

Figure 5–31 (FSB–36). Mesangio-capillary sclerosis with proliferation and deposits. Note the thickened GBM's, mesangial hypercellularity, and deposits within the GBM as well as on its endothelial aspect. The mesangial region also contains deposits.

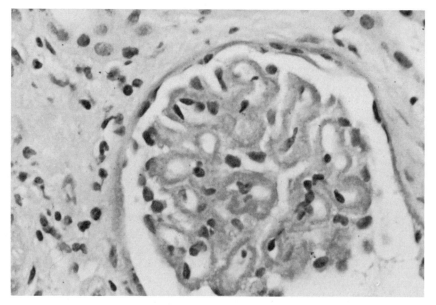

Figure 5–32 (FSB–37). Advanced membranous glomerulonephritis: glomerulus with uniformly and diffusely thickened basement membranes. Note the relative hypocellularity of the glomerulus. There is marked interstitial fibrosis and loss of tubular architecture in the surrounding parenchyma.

5–17a, b, c; Figure 5–32, FSB–37). The capillary spaces are widely patent and there appears to be a decrease in the total number of cells in the tufts. With higher resolution the basement membrane thickening may be seen to be composed of spikes of basement membrane material projecting toward the epithelial cells, which have fused foot processes. Between the spikes are deposits of electron-dense material which may be seen by immunofluorescence staining to contain gamma-globulin. Thus, the epithelial surface of the GBM has a comb-like appearance. The significance or pathogenesis of this change is unclear. As in the proliferative form of chronic GN, the tubular, interstitial, and vascular changes reflect the state of the disease and level and duration of hypertension.

The membranous form of CGN is much less common than the proliferative variety. Since the most prominent change initially noted was diffusely thickened glomerular basement membranes, it was called membranous glomerulonephritis. This lesion does not appear to be inflammatory and, therefore, the term glomerulonephr*itis* is not entirely appropriate. The name "membranous glomerulonephritis" however, is deeply ingrained in textbooks and journals and will likely persist. As

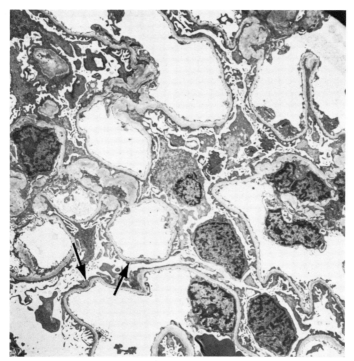

Figure 5–33 (FSB–38).   Nephrotic syndrome and fusion of pedicels. Electron micrograph of a peripheral capillary loop with fusion of epithelial foot processes (arrows). No other abnormalities are shown.

in the other forms of chronic renal disease, presumably primarily glomerular in origin, we know nothing of its etiology. However, serial renal biopsy studies of this form of disease suggest that it progresses by a gradual increase in the amount of glomerular basement membrane material so that the "teeth" tend to fuse and the deposits disappear. The mesangial regions also thicken, and eventually the blood supply to the tufts disappears and the glomerulus becomes obsolescent. This process appears to require a number of years from beginning to end.

Recently there has been described another form of chronic renal disease primarily affecting the glomerulus. It is histologically characterized by thickened glomerular basement membranes, mesangial hypercellularity, and deposits. The GBM's contain deposits within their substance or on the endothelial side. The presence of deposits within the thickened GBM's gives them the appearance of being split or duplicated (Fig. 5–31). The deposits contain complement components and IgG singly or in combination. The clinical findings are usually those of the nephrotic syndrome. Since the initial patients with this picture were found to have hypocomplementemia, it was called hypocomplementemic GN. This name has been dropped, since many patients do not have depressed serum complement levels and since hypocomplementemia occurs in a multitude of other diseases. Since the histologic picture is reasonably distinct, it has been called membrano-proliferative or mesangio-capillary GN. The sclerosis gradually increases over a period of years, although the exact time varies from 3 to over 10 years. No therapy has thus far proven effective.

Proliferative and Sclerosing Chronic GN with a Lobular Configuration. This is a relatively uncommon form of glomerular lesion which, like the proliferative variety, may show focal areas of basement membrane thickening. The feature which differentiates this form from the other two is that the mesangial proliferation and sclerosis have altered the glomerular architecture so that the tufts appear to be compressed together into lobules. The only other condition with which this may be confused is that seen with diabetes mellitus. However, in the later stages of diabetes mellitus, large acellular nodules are seen in the mesangial regions, and the glomerular basement membranes are usually *diffusely* thickened.

Diabetic Glomerulosclerosis. As the name implies, the histologic lesion is one of sclerosis (or scarring) of the glomeruli. Prominent vascular, tubular, and interstitial changes are also present. The characteristic feature is an increase in extracellular material leading to thickened basement membranes (glomerular, tubular, and vascular). In the glomeruli this is so pronounced that nodules of extracellular material accumulate in the mesangial regions (p. 194).

Renal failure is often signalled by the onset of hypertension or the nephrotic syndrome. Hypertension is more often seen in those patients

who have had no or only trace proteinuria and in whom chronic proliferative GN is detected histologically.

Nephrotic Syndrome (NS)

The nephrotic syndrome is defined as a composite of characteristic
clinical and laboratory findings consisting of proteinuria (>2 gm/m^2/24
hrs), edema, hypoalbuminemia, and hyperlipidemia. In previous sections of this chapter renal reactions to injury and a few illustrative
diseases have been presented. Most have had substantial glomerular involvement. The nephrotic syndrome may be associated with any of the
general reactions, from the most difficult to detect through almost
complete renal destruction, although the most common in adults are
those associated with sclerosis (membranous and diabetic). By way of
contrast, the most common glomerular lesion in the NS of childhood can
be recognized only by electron microscopy (fusion of the pedicels) (Figure 5–33, FSB–38). Clearly, the NS does not respect anatomic boundaries. Because the exact type of renal disease may vary widely, there is
clinical significance in determining the underlying disease process in the
patient with NS. As stated in previous sections, the *histologic picture* is
most important in determining the type, distribution, and severity of the
renal abnormalities and determining the prognosis. The *diagnosis* is
made clinically. The renal lesions of SLE and the NS best illustrate this
principle since the diagnosis, established by other means, prompts a
biopsy to determine the exact pathologic process.

The NS of children and that of adults differ in the incidence of associated renal lesions. In childhood the NS commonly has no or minimal
associated histologic renal change, while in adults there is anatomic evidence of underlying disease. The following discussion will consider
mainly the *childhood* form of the *nephrotic syndrome* with no associated
light microscopic lesion. Many other adjectives are used, such as lipoid
or idiopathic nephrosis. Although this condition has been known and
studied for many years, it is poorly understood. Age and sex play some
role in its pathogenesis, for the majority of cases occur between the ages
of 18 months and 10 years and there is a predominance of males. In the
nephrotic syndrome of childhood no histological changes are seen by
light microscopy, but electron microscopic examination reveals fusion of
the foot processes of the glomerular epithelial cells. When the nephrotic
syndrome occurs during the *first year of life*, it is usually a more severe
disease and ends fatally in the overwhelming majority of cases (see p.
178).

In the clinical approach to the nephrotic syndrome it is important to
determine which histologic changes are present, in order that appropriate treatment may be employed and some estimation of prognosis established. The use of renal biopsy has helped in differentiating those

cases of nephrotic syndrome associated with fixed renal disease from those without light microscopic change. Those factors other than histologic appearance which are helpful in establishing the diagnosis of idiopathic NS are:

(1) Normal renal function
(2) Urine sediment containing only renal cells or renal cell casts (oval fat bodies are tubular cells containing lipid)
(3) Absence of hypertension
(4) Low molecular weight proteinuria
(5) Remission of proteinuria with steroid therapy.

The overall survival rate in the childhood nephrotic syndrome is said to be 60 to 75 per cent, but most studies include patients who may have had the nephrotic syndrome associated with glomerulonephritis or other systemic diseases. The survival rate of children, over one year of age, with this minimal lesion form of the nephrotic syndrome is thought to be considerably higher (95 per cent) if they could be separated from all those associated with other types of renal disease.

The nephrotic syndrome in *adults* may occur in the absence of significant histologic renal abnormalities, and in this form the prognosis and response to therapy are identical to that seen in children. However, more frequently an adult with the nephrotic syndrome has histologic evidence of glomerular cell proliferation or glomerular sclerosis. In this instance, as with children, the symptoms and signs are quite often glucocorticoid resistant, that is, steroids may reduce the proteinuria but continual glucocorticoid therapy is required to keep the proteinuria at a low level. Other anti-inflammatory agents such as azathioprine and cyclophosphamide are now being used as an adjunct to, or in place of, glucocorticoids.

In summary, both the juvenile and adult forms of the nephrotic syndrome may be associated with a varied pathologic picture corresponding to the primary disease process (minimal change, glomerulonephritis, diabetes, or other process). The nephrotic syndrome adds nothing more to the histologic findings of the primary disease than large numbers of hyaline casts and desquamated, fat-filled columnar epithelial cells within tubular lumens.

The congenital nephrotic syndrome is so titled in order to stress the difference existing between this condition and the nephrotic syndrome of childhood. Several factors suggest that the disease has its onset during intra-uterine life. The disease is always fatal. The longest survival has been 3 years. Most patients die with secondary infections in spite of normal renal function. Treatment with glucocorticoids has been of no value. The immunosuppressive drugs have not been given a full therapeutic trial, but initial observations suggest that they, too, will be of little value. The histologic changes are varied. The majority of cases show only dilatation of the tubules.

Tubular Diseases

The final composition and volume of the bladder urine is dependent on the cells of each region of the nephron. This requires that the appropriate metabolic processes be intact and complete in each cell, that filtrate be delivered at an appropriate rate, and that the interstitial and vascular compartments be able to deliver nutrients or substances to be secreted to the cell and carry away reabsorbed materials and metabolites. Since the total number of nephrons greatly exceeds that required to maintain adequate renal function, to become clinically apparent a lesion must involve either a substantial number of the total nephrons or an isolated metabolic step in a specific segment. These are clinically apparent as two quite different disease processes. The first is commonly called *tubular necrosis*, but the term *tubular injury* is preferred since frank necrosis is uncommon. Tubular function is impaired in affected nephrons in proportion to the degree of structural damage. It often presents as acute renal failure because the tubular damage is diffuse. The disease is transient with recovery in most patients who are kept alive with dialysis and do not die from other causes. By way of contrast, the second type presents as a functional tubular disorder which is persistent and isolated with impairment of *specific* functions. These are rare but physiologically instructive diseases, and they will be briefly considered.

TUBULAR INJURY is the most common cause of acute renal failure. Other causes are severe glomerulonephritis, renal cortical necrosis, and acute bilateral vascular or ureteral obstruction. The two main causes of tubular injury are: (1) ischemia with anoxic tubular damage, and (2) necrosis of the tubular epithelial cells mediated by toxins which act directly on specific cells or specific subcellular organelles. The former is most commonly associated with prolonged hypotension (shock), such as that accompanying crush injuries, major operative procedures in high-risk patients, traumatic injuries, septicemia, or burns. Substances producing nephrotoxic damage have been discussed in Chapter 3. The clinical manifestations of acute renal failure can be divided into four phases: (1) prodromal, (2) anuria or oliguria, (3) diuresis, and (4) recovery. The prodromal phase varies in duration, depending upon causative factors such as the dosage of toxin ingested or the duration and severity of hypotension. The *anuric or oliguric phase* is defined by loss of nephron function, as exhibited by a urine volume of less than 500 ml daily (less than 20 ml/hr), a concentrating defect manifested by a urine to plasma osmolality ratio of 0.9 to 1.1, and a rising plasma creatinine. Although oliguria is the sign most frequently sought in the early recognition of this problem, it is of interest that approximately 20 per cent of patients with tubular injury never manifest oliguria although a concentrating defect and steadily increasing azotemia are always present. Acute renal failure in diffuse tubular injury may be associated with water excess and increasing concentrations of metabolites, electrolytes, and administered drugs unless preventative measures are instituted as soon as the problem is recognized. Hyperkalemia is particularly dangerous and may produce fatal arrhythmias unless corrected promptly. The use of good parenteral or oral nutrition coupled with early adequate dialysis has decreased mortality during this stage and prevented such complications. The oliguric phase may last from hours to weeks, depending upon the cause. A renal biopsy is often performed at this point to determine the site of the lesion producing anuria or oliguria and its potential reversibility.

The *diuretic phase* is quite important, since mismanagement may cause the death of the patient. During this period urine flow again begins, but inadequate tubular regeneration plus interstitial edema and inflammation prevent normal renal function. The urine is similar to an ultrafiltrate of plasma, and large quantities of electrolytes and water may be lost. Although the urine volume may be high, the excretion of urea and creatinine is so low that their plasma levels continue to rise or only fall very slowly. The duration of this phase is variable but approximates 5 to 7 days. The *recovery phase* is characterized by return of tubular function with electrolyte and water conservation, with a subsequent drop in

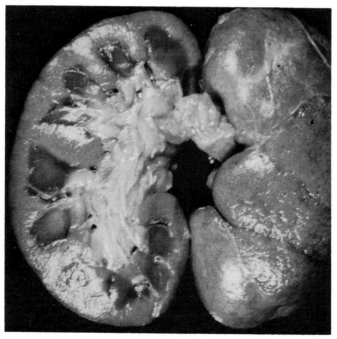

Figure 5–34 (FSB–39). Renal failure with diffuse necrosis: gross photograph of a kidney with a relatively pale cortex and dark papillae. The patient ingested "pine-oil" disinfectant. The kidney weighed 600 gm.

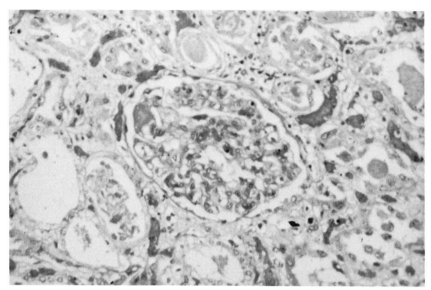

Figure 5–35 (FSB–40). Tubular necrosis: light micrograph from same patient as Figure 5–34, showing necrosis of nearly all tubular segments. Note the cellular debris within the tubular lumina, consisting of degenerating cells and laked protein.

urine volume, and with a decreasing azotemia. Although renal function may not return entirely to normal in all patients, a slow improvement in GFR and concentrating capacity continues for several months after the onset of diuresis.

Grossly the kidneys are large and swollen, and have a soft consistency. The cortex is pale and the medulla is often quite dark (Figure 5–34, FSB–39). Microscopically the glomeruli are normal. The tubules may show a variety of changes depending on the phase in which the biopsy is done (Figure 5–35, FSB–40). Evidence of necrosis is not frequently seen, and when present is very patchy in distribution. The proximal tubules are frequently dilated, containing protein, desquamated cells, and debris. It is thought that this material (in the form of casts) obstructs the tubules, leading to impairment of flow, back diffusion of tubular fluid and, therefore, oliguria. Later in the disease the lining cells may be seen to be flattened and to contain mitotic figures. Changes in the loop of Henle and distal or collecting tubules are not consistent and are thought to be due to the casts found in their lumina. The interstitium is edematous, and this may be the most prominent feature (Figure 5–36, FSB–41). Inflammatory cells of all varieties are frequently found in tubules and the interstitium.

In the older literature, tubular necrosis was thought to be predominantly in the distal tubule, and the condition was labeled lower nephron nephrosis. Nephron dissection studies, however, pinpoint lesions both at

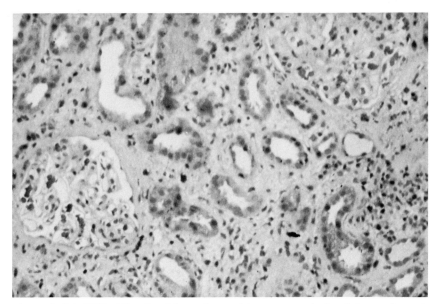

Figure 5–36 (FSB–41). In this patient with severe tubular injury, there is marked interstitial filtrate and edema. Few proximal tubular profiles are apparent.

the lower end of the proximal tubules and at the distal convoluted tubule.

Persistent Disorders of Tubular Function. Most diseases affecting the kidney impair all aspects of function to some degree. There are, however, a group of diseases exhibiting a primary disturbance of tubular function with GFR remaining near normal. These diseases are congenital and acquired defects of specific regulatory function of the kidney which may occur either singly or in specific constellations reflecting the functional anatomy of the tubules. The following brief discussion of a few tubular disorders will point out the pathophysiologic process involved. They are conveniently divided into: (1) proximal tubular and (2) distal tubular and collecting duct disorders.

Proximal Tubular Disorders. The wide range of defects which may occur as a result of proximal tubular damage or dysfunction is not surprising in view of the multiple functions of this structure. *Renal glycosuria* is a benign congenital condition in which there is an unusually low transport maximum for glucose reabsorption. Its chief importance is that it may mistakenly lead to the diagnosis of diabetes mellitus. *Renal phosphaturia* may occur alone or in combination with other defects. The excessive excretion of phosphate is associated with poor bone formation and resistance to ordinary doses of vitamin D. *The Fanconi syndrome* is the eponym applied to conditions in which several proximal tubular functions are disturbed. The pattern varies, but in most cases the clearance and excretion of several amino acids is high. This is referred to as a generalized aminoaciduria in order to distinguish it from the large group of genetic diseases in which specific amino acids are excreted in large quantities because of their overproduction. Patients with the Fanconi syndrome not only have aminoaciduria but often have phosphaturia, high clearance of uric acid, and wastage of calcium. *Proximal renal tubular acidosis* may occur as part of the Fanconi syndrome or by itself. The pathophysiology of this disorder is related to a reduced transport of bicarbonate ion (Chapter 4).

Distal Tubular and Collecting Duct Defects. This area of the nephron is primarily responsible for the development of a large hydrogen ion gradient and concentration of the urine. *Distal renal tubular acidosis* is a defect in renal acidification and has been discussed previously (Chapter 4). It may be a congenital defect or may be acquired in the course of diseases such as pyelonephritis, papillary necrosis, and cirrhosis. These same patients may also have mild defects in concentrating capacity. More severe water wastage occurs among a group of children with *renal diabetes insipidus* who have a specific defect in the responsiveness of the collecting duct to ADH, thus preventing renal production of an isotonic or hypertonic urine.

ARTERIAL AND ARTERIOLAR DISEASE OF THE KIDNEY INCLUDING HYPERTENSION

The vessels of the kidney are exposed to a high and relatively constant blood flow. In common with all muscular arteries, their main function is the transmission and distribution of blood. There is also a small but definite transport of nutrients from the intima to the adventitia. The volume and composition of the material which gains access to the vascular wall from the lumen depend on the integrity of the endothelium.

Arteries have a relatively limited response to injury. If the endothelium is injured, by deposition of antigen-antibody complexes or thrombi, plasma proteins and cellular elements gain access to the vascular wall. The result initially is fibrin formation. If the insult is severe, thrombosis may result. Proliferation of intimal cells follows more mild or chronic injury. If the injury continues and intimal proliferation persists, extracellular material is laid down between the cells to form multiple layers of the internal elastic membrane. These apparently reduce the distensibility of the vessels as well as their luminal size. Relatively little is known about the responses of the media to injury. In the presence of a continuously elevated blood pressure there appears to be hypertrophy of the smooth muscle cells, and fibrosis of this layer has been described in recipients of renal allografts.

Deposits of amorphous material (hyaline) are seen beneath the intimal cells and in the media of vessels in a variety of patients. This material contains various serum proteins and fragments of degenerated cells. It is presumed to be the result of excessive filtration and deposition of plasma proteins.

Abnormally high blood pressure is often associated with diseases of the renal vessels. The exact relationships are not understood, for one can occur without the other. Hypertension, especially if sustained, may cause disease of the vessels, and there are situations (relatively infrequent) in which vascular disease appears to cause or perpetuate hypertension. For these reasons, hypertension and vascular disease of the kidney are considered together.

Vascular disease of the kidney associated with hypertension can be divided into five types.

1. *Arteriosclerosis* (frequently called *atherosclerosis*) primarily affects the larger renal vessels and is a part of a generalized atherosclerotic process. It thus is common in the older age groups. The vessel becomes sclerotic and less resilient in this degenerative process (Figure 5–37, FSB–42; Figure 5–38), and the cross-sectional area of the lumen is decreased.

Arteriosclerosis frequently occurs in the absence of elevated blood pressure, but the process is generally thought to be accelerated by hypertension. Occasionally an atherosclerotic plaque in a major blood vessel

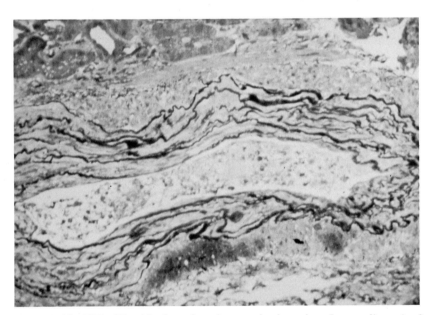

Figure 5–37 (FSB–42). Nephrosclerosis: an elastic stain of a medium-sized vessel. The elastica is stained black and can be seen to be multi-layered on the intimal side of the media.

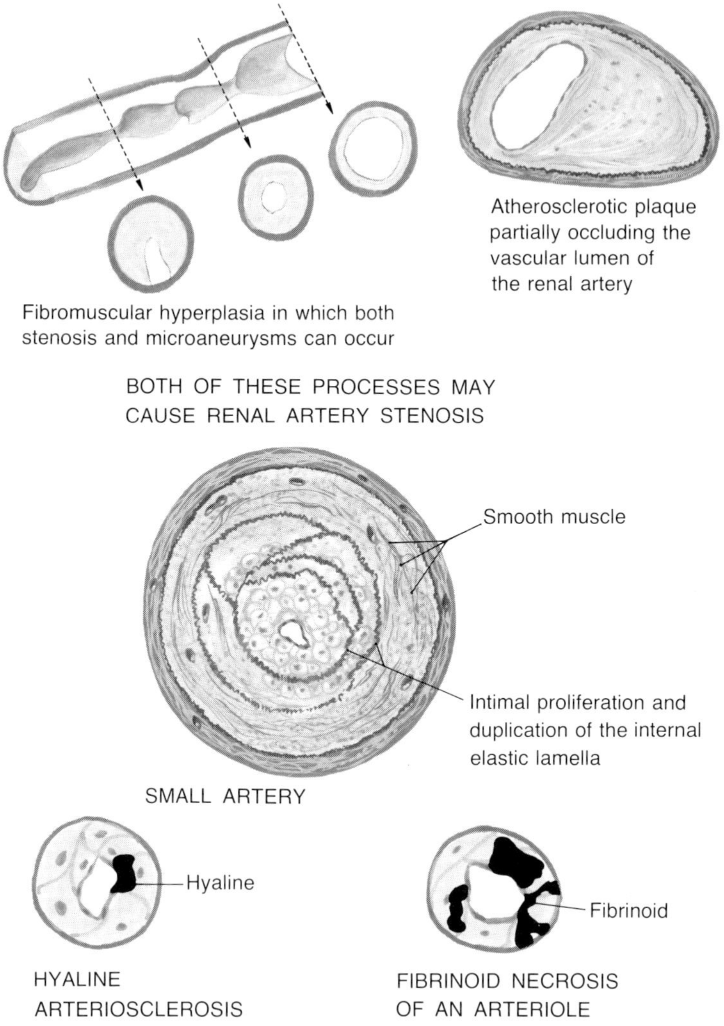

Atherosclerotic plaque
partially occluding the
vascular lumen of
the renal artery

Fibromuscular hyperplasia in which both
stenosis and microaneurysms can occur

BOTH OF THESE PROCESSES MAY
CAUSE RENAL ARTERY STENOSIS

Smooth muscle

Intimal proliferation and
duplication of the internal
elastic lamella

SMALL ARTERY

Hyaline

Fibrinoid

HYALINE   FIBRINOID NECROSIS
ARTERIOSCLEROSIS   OF AN ARTERIOLE

Figure 5–38.   Arteriosclerosis causing stenosis of renal artery.

may reduce renal blood flow enough to cause renovascular hypertension (Figure 5–39, FSB–43).

2. *Arteriolar nephrosclerosis* is the term used to describe changes in renal arterioles thought to be related to arteriosclerosis. It is often seen in association with prolonged hypertension. It may also occur in the absence of elevated blood pressure, especially in diabetics. A deposit of hyaline material (staining a homogeneous light pink with hemotoxylin and eosin) (Figure 5–40, FSB–44; Figure 5–38) or intimal proliferation, or both, may be seen.

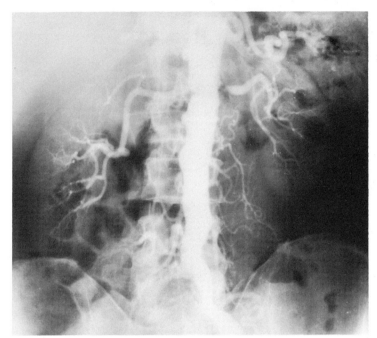

Figure 5-39 (FSB-43). Atherosclerotic renal artery stenosis: marked athero-sclerotic changes throughout the aorta, with narrowing of left renal artery at its takeoff from the aorta.

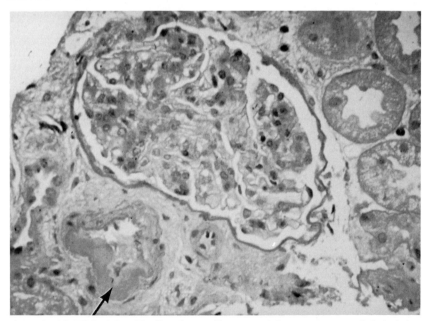

Figure 5-40 (FSB-44). Hyaline in small artery. A homogeneous pink-staining material can be seen in the wall of the small artery in the lower left corner (arrow). This material appears to lie in the region of the media.

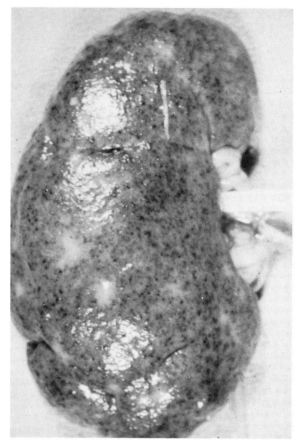

Figure 5–41 (FSB–45). Multiple petechial hemorrhages. This is a kidney from a patient with accelerated hypertension. The multiple punctate hemorrhagic spots on the cortex alternate with pale ischemic areas. The hemorrhages correspond to areas of severe vascular damage.

3. *Proliferative endarteritis* means intimal proliferation primarily involving small arteries of the kidney, such as the arcuate or intralobar branches. This is an unusual process most commonly associated with severe (often called *malignant*) hypertension or with renal transplant rejection. Grossly the kidneys are large and have a cortical petechia (Figure 5–41, FSB–45). Microscopically there is marked thickening of small arterial walls due to myointimal cell proliferation, and fine concentric layering of elastic fibers leading to a virtual obliteration of the vascular lumen (Figure 5–38; Figure 5–42, FSB–46).

4. *Fibrinoid necrosis,* also involving the arterioles, usually the afferent, is the anatomical correlate of severe hypertension (Figure 5–38; Figure 5–43, FSB–47). It differs from proliferative endarteritis not only

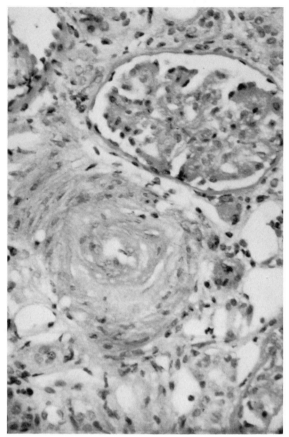

Figure 5–42 (FSB–46). Proliferative end-arteritis. Internal to the media of this small artery there is marked proliferation of cells and deposition of extra-cellular material. The vascular lumen is severely compromised. Note that the glomerulus at the upper right appears shrunken and hypocellular.

in appearance but also in that it involves only arterioles. It consists of four basic processes: (1) necrosis of muscle fibers, (2) infiltration of media and intima with plasma proteins and often red blood cells (the fibrinoid material is due to plasma proteins which give the lesion a very characteristic, intensely bright staining, pink, granular quality on hemotoxylin and eosin staining), (3) an inflammatory cell infiltrate, and (4) proliferation of myointimal cells. These lesions often lead to complete obliteration of the vessel.

5. *Fibromuscular hyperplasia* affecting the main renal artery or its principal branches is a disease presenting in early adulthood as a cause of renovascular hypertension. Younger women are affected more commonly than men. The lesion is characterized by rings of hyperplasia of the muscular elements of the media of the renal arteries, with alternating zones of medial destruction and atrophy resulting in what are actu-

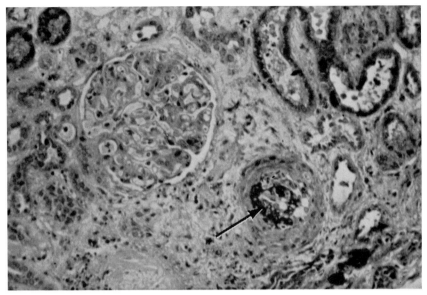

Figure 5–43 (FSB–47). Fibrin in a vessel wall. In this patient with accelerated hypertension, fibrinoid (arrow) can be seen within the proliferating cells in the zone between the media and the lumen. This is so-called fibrinoid necrosis.

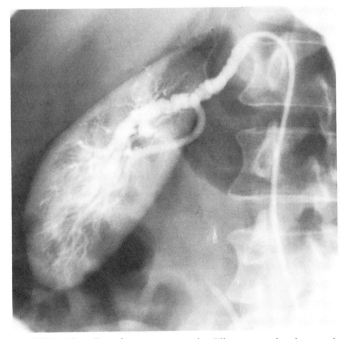

Figure 5–44 (FSB–48). Renal artery stenosis. Fibromuscular hyperplasia producing hypertension as a result of narrowing of renal artery in a young woman.

ally mural microaneurysms. Functionally this results in stenosis and peculiar beaded appearance, best seen on arteriography. Both renal vessels are frequently involved (Figure 5–44, FSB–48).

Any of these vascular diseases associated with ischemia can lead to glomerular sclerosis and interstitial fibrosis with concomitant reduction of renal function. Early in the development of glomerular sclerosis, there is shrinkage of the glomerular tuft, wrinkling and thickening of the glomerular basement membrane, and deposition of collagen. In the latest stages, the glomeruli remain only as shrunken GBM's surrounded by a dense mass of collagen. During the evolution of this process, the interstitium and tubules usually become atrophic and sclerotic. The important clinical conditions which may be associated with these pathological changes are reviewed below.

TYPES OF HYPERTENSION

Essential hypertension is the condition in which the blood pressure is raised for no single, clear reason. The vast majority of people with hypertension fall into this category. It is a continuum starting with those people who are in every sense healthy, have no clinical or anatomic evidence of end organ damage, a blood pressure only slightly elevated above an arbitrary upper limit of normal (normal: 160/90), and a prognosis for a life span equal or nearly equal to the one without an elevated blood pressure. At the other end of the spectrum are patients with severe hypertension, renal failure, an enlarged heart, vascular disease of the brain, and prospects for an early death. The etiology of hypertension in any group is unclear; there is probably not a single, simple cause. Genetic predisposition, stress of life, obesity, dietary sodium ingestion, and personality have all been identified as contributing factors. Certain groups of people have been identified as statistically more likely to have an unfavorable course. They should, therefore, be treated. For example, those with enlarged hearts, renal failure, or hypertensive retinopathy should be treated more vigorously than those with no changes. There is recent evidence that those patients with high renin levels are more likely to develop complications than those with low renin levels. Even among this latter group (the benign hypertensive), it is generally recognized that the young black male is far more likely to develop "malignant" hypertension than the elderly obese white female with the same blood pressure. The causes of early death are stroke, heart disease (myocardial infarction and congestive heart failure), and renal failure. About 5 per cent of patients with essential hypertension enter the malignant phase and, as noted, certain patients are more likely than others to develop this complication. The renal lesion most commonly noted in association with essential hypertension is *arteriolar nephrosclerosis*.

Malignant or accelerated hypertension is that clinical condition in which blood pressure rises rapidly over the course of months, weeks, or even days. At this point, the patient usually complains of headaches and visual disturbances, and has a very high blood pressure. Funduscopic examination reveals hemorrhages, exudates, and papilledema. Renal function fails rapidly. Histologically there is fibrinoid necrosis involving first arterioles, then glomeruli, and finally the whole vasculature. This rapidly progressive injury is directly related to the level of blood pressure and constitutes the major cause of death in this group. The process can be halted by rapid control of blood pressure using potent antihypertensive drugs. Renal function seldom returns to normal since the fibrinoid necrosis results in scarring and in permanent loss of the affected nephrons. Similar vascular lesions are seen in other organs. Cerebrovascular accidents, myocardial infarction or congestive heart failure, hemorrhagic strokes, and brain infarctions, in addition to renal disease, may cause early death. Because most hypertension is "essential," the majority of those who develop malignant hypertension are from this group. However, other forms of hypertension, especially renovascular, may lead to malignant hypertension. Regardless of the original cause of the blood pressure elevation, the unique feature of malignant hypertension is its self-perpetuating character unless early, aggressive therapy is instituted. The mechanism is presumably the damage to the afferent arterioles of the glomeruli.

Renal artery stenosis with partial occlusion of the renal artery to one or both kidneys is a cause of hypertension in 5 to 10% of the hypertensive population. It is noteworthy that renal artery stenosis may exist without the presence of hypertension, and some patients may have both stenosis and hypertension without there being a causal relationship. The latter condition is particularly true among older patients whose arterial obstruction is usually caused by arteriosclerosis, which is the commonest cause of arterial obstruction in this age group. In younger patients with hypertension, especially women, renal artery stenosis is more commonly caused by fibromuscular hyperplasia.

Partial obstruction of the main renal artery or of smaller branches apparently produces hypertension by way of the renin-angiotensin-aldosterone mechanism (see Chapter 2). Activation of this mechanism is caused by a reduction in blood flow and/or pressure, which produces renin release with resultant increase in angiotensin II and aldosterone. Correction of the vascular lesion or removal of the affected kidney will often lower the blood pressure. However, renovascular hypertension of long duration causes secondary vascular changes in the "normal" contralateral kidney, and hypertension may persist after surgical correction of the stenotic area. In a few cases it has been necessary to remove a "normal" kidney (with secondary small vessel disease secondary to hypertension) after repairing the large vessel blood supply to the ischemic kidney (whose small vessels are normal, having been protected from the effects of the hypertension by the main artery lesion). Renovascular hypertension of long duration may also cause fixed secondary changes in the control of blood pressure.

Primary aldosteronism is a condition causing relatively mild hypertension, seldom progressing to malignant hypertension. It results from autonomous secretion of aldosterone by small benign tumors (adenomas) or diffuse hyperplasia of the adrenal cortex. Because secretion occurs autonomously, the normal feedback mechanism operates to reduce the secretion of renin. Renin levels are therefore characteristically low in this disease. Blood pressure is increased, presumably because of sodium retention caused by the hypersecretion of aldosterone. The resulting increase in total body sodium raises the ECV, reduces the vascular compliance, and increases peripheral resistance, thereby raising blood pressure. Because of an escape mechanism associated with a decreasing renal sodium retention, edema is rarely produced.

Primary aldosteronism not only causes the retention of sodium, but also causes the renal wastage of potassium and hydrogen, which may lead to a mild hypokalemia and metabolic alkalosis. For this reason, hypertensive patients with a low serum potassium or a high serum bicar-

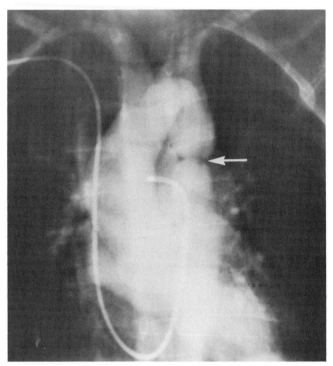

Figure 5–45 (FSB–49). Coarctation of aorta: aortogram showing stenosis (arrow) in descending portion of aortic arch.

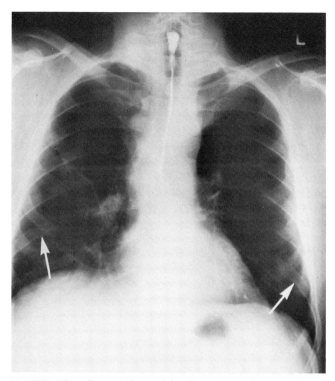

Figure 5–46 (FSB–50). Coarctation, with rib notching (arrows) from collateral circulation showing in the lower margin of ribs.

bonate who are not in the accelerated phase of hypertension or taking diuretics should be suspected of having an adrenal tumor (or tumors) secreting aldosterone. The distinction between primary and secondary aldosteronism with hypertension is usually based on a renin determination (high in secondary and low in primary aldosteronism).

Coarctation of the aorta is often found early in life (Figure 5–45, FSB–49). However, the patients, especially males, may be perfectly healthy until the third decade of life or even later. The diagnosis should always be considered when hypertension is present. It may be ruled out by simultaneous palpation of the femoral and radial pulses, looking for a delay in the femoral pulse; and by a reduction of blood pressure in the legs as compared to the arms (normally 20 mm Hg higher in the leg). If coarctation is suspected, corroboration is sought from a chest film, which will usually demonstrate typical rib "notching" (Figure 5–46, FSB–50). The notching is due to erosion of the inferior surface of the rib by the greatly dilated intercostal arteries, which are supplying oxygenated blood to the lower body distal to the coarctation. Final diagnosis is by aortography, and surgical repair is a well-established procedure. Renal vessels are usually spared in this condition, since the coarctation usually appears in the thoracic aorta.

Pheochromocytoma is an extremely rare cause of hypertension. This is a tumor of ectodermal origin, arising in the adrenal medulla or the glands of Zuckerkandl, which secrete epinephrine or norepinephrine. Although the hypertension may be periodic, it is often sustained. The patient has symptoms of episodic palpitations, pallor, vague abdominal pain, and perspiration (the four p's). Diagnosis is made by measurement of catecholamines in plasma or urine, during periods of elevated blood pressure.

Pyelonephritis and hypertension are frequently seen in the same patient. However, it rarely can be demonstrated that a unilaterally pyelonephritic kidney is actually causing the hypertension. This is not too surprising, since the total renal parenchyma, including the JGA, is destroyed in this disease. More common is the small atrophic or hypoplastic kidney, whose removal results in a return to normal blood pressure.

Systemic illness, in which hypertension is seen or may be a prominent feature, seldom if ever presents a problem of differential diagnosis. The therapy of hypertension in association with adrenal cortical hyperfunction (Cushing's syndrome) is that of the primary disease. Similarly, the hypertension in association with polyarteritis nodosa and systemic lupus erythematosus is best treated medically and may improve if the basic process can be controlled. As previously noted, hypertension may be a complication of advanced renal failure. Rigid sodium restriction usually reduces the blood pressure in hypertension without regard to the primary disease.

MORPHOLOGY AND CLINICAL DISORDERS OF THE KIDNEY RELATED TO DIABETES

Renal disease has become an increasingly common problem among diabetics as their life expectancy increases with the use of insulin and other modalities of therapy. The renal disease takes several forms which can co-exist.

Diabetic glomerulosclerosis is the best known and most specific lesion. It is usually progressive over many years, and therefore the kidney may at one time appear normal, another time swollen, and in its last stages, small and scarred. Histologically, there is hyaline thickening of the glomerular basement membrane and the mesangial regions of the glomerular tuft. This thickening may be diffuse or nodular (Figure 5–47, FSB–51). The nodular diabetic glomerulosclerosis is the most pathognomonic histological change of diabetes. As these changes progress, the glomeruli may become obsolescent, the tubules atrophic, and the interstitium fibrotic, just as they do in other degenerative diseases of the kid-

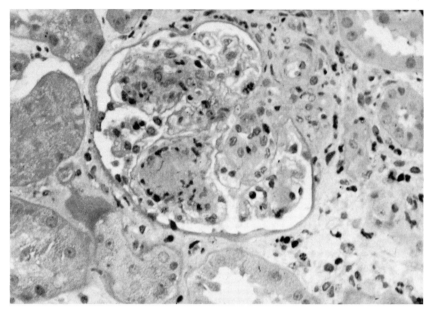

Figure 5-47 (FSB-51). Diabetic glomerulosclerosis. The glomerular basement membranes are diffusely thickened and the mesangial regions contain large amorphous masses of hyalin material, which is devoid of cells.

ney such as sclerosing glomerulonephritis, hypertension, persistent infection, stone formation, and obstruction.

Atherosclerosis and *arteriolosclerosis* are very common among diabetics and may further damage the kidney. Occasionally, papillary necrosis occurs in diabetics, perhaps because of the combination of degenerative vascular disease and infection.

As a result of these changes, progressive renal failure may be seen. There is little evidence that better control of blood sugar with insulin decreases the rate of progression. In addition, and for reasons that are unclear, diabetics develop the nephrotic syndrome, which is often particularly difficult to manage. Often they have some degree of concomitant renal failure.

INTERSTITIAL DISEASES

Up to this point, we have discussed processes which affect the glomeruli, the vessels, and the tubules of the kidney. There are also diseases which appear primarily to affect the fourth compartment, the interstitium. Bear in mind that as glomerulonephritis, hypertensive vascular disease, diabetes, and other diseases progress, the interstitium becomes fibrotic. The severity of the interstitial fibrosis, regardless of its cause, correlates quite well with changes in renal function.

Pyelonephritis (infection of the kidney) is mentioned here as one of the causes of interstitial inflammation or fibrosis. *Acute pyelonephritis* is characterized by patchy infiltration of the interstitium (particularly in the medulla) by neutrophils, lymphocytes, and plasma cells. Unless the infection is hematogenously disseminated, abscesses or bacteria are seldom seen. Bacteria usually reach the kidney by way of the collecting system. *Chronic pyelonephritis* causes patchy areas of fibrosis which may become confluent. Bacteria are seldom seen.

Fibrosis and infiltration of the interstitium by chronic inflammation cells is certainly not a specific finding, yet the diagnosis of *"chronic pyelonephritis"* has often been made on the basis of this histologic finding alone. We are becoming aware, however, that other conditions associated with destruction of renal parenchyma may lead to an identical appearance. The analgesic abuse syndrome appears to be a relatively frequent cause of diffuse interstitial nephritis. This syndrome, first reported among adults consuming huge quantities of phenacetin, aspirin, and caffeine in Europe, is now being seen with increasing frequency in America. The lesion is apparently caused by degeneration of the medullary vasae rectae. In its final stages, the medullary pyramids may become necrotic and slough off (*papillary necrosis*) (Figure 5–48, FSB–52). Its pathophysiology and the role of these various drugs is not clearly understood. *Gout* which is associated with *hyperuricemia* may also

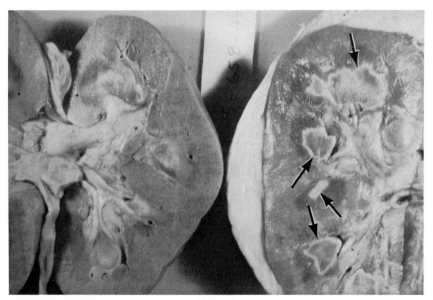

Figure 5–48 (FSB–52). Papillary necrosis. The papillae on the right are a white color and are sharply marginated from the normal pink renal parenchyma. The white areas represent necrosis (arrows). Compare them with the papillae on the left, which are only partially involved.

lead to interstitial fibrosis apparently caused by the deposition of urate crystals in the tubules, leading to an inflammatory response and fibrosis. While seeing the crystals microscopically might aid in the interpretation of the lesion, they are not always visible.

CORTICAL NECROSIS

Cortical necrosis is the result of a sudden, usually catastrophic loss of circulating blood to the kidney. It may involve the entire kidney or only a small part of it. Thrombosis or embolism to the renal artery or one of its main branches may be the cause. Extremely severe trauma, burns, or bleeding may also cause cortical necrosis, though more commonly the reversible renal disease called acute tubular necrosis results. However, the most common cause is related to pregnancy. Both septic abortion and abruptio placentae (premature separation of the placenta) appear to trigger a complex set of enzymatic conversions of both vasoactive polypeptides and clotting factor, leading to massive intravascular clotting analogous to the experimental Shwartzman's phenomenon. Cortical necrosis is, of course, irreversible, because the damage is so extensive.

END-STAGE KIDNEY DISEASE

The term *end-stage renal disease* was coined by clinicians to describe the condition resulting from slowly progressive renal failure. Strictly speaking, end-stage renal disease exists whenever the kidney has sustained enough damage to cease functioning permanently. This would include many diseases which have a very short clinical course, but the term is not used in these conditions. As in previous sections, it is again clear that the current nomenclature obscures rather than clarifies the basic anatomic, physiological, or clinical facts.

Common to all conditions considered in the category of end-stage renal disease is the fact that the number of functioning nephrons is diminished over a prolonged time span. The exact causes are quite diverse, but again one can make some order of the chaos by subdividing them into the basic anatomic segments. Therefore, the following discussion will consider first glomerular diseases and then vascular diseases. It is well to keep in mind that, while these general subdivisions can be made, by the time renal failure ensues all compartments are affected quite severely and the physician may have to use a crystal ball to arrive at the "correct diagnosis." It is also possible that in the frenzy to make a diagnosis we ignore the fact that all of the components of the kidney are involved in most diseases and that artificial boundaries have no real meaning.

Chronic Renal Disease Presumed to Be Primarily Glomerular.
As physicians gather around the autopsy table or the x-ray view box con-
templating bilaterally small kidneys, primary glomerular disease is the
most frequently considered diagnosis. While these observers may be correct, there is little evidence to support that stand. The antecedent stages,
to say nothing of the etiologic factors, have never been adequately studied. Most of the information published about this phase of renal disease
has been taken from autopsy series. It is quite clear that from this type of
information, one can never understand the evolution of the process
(since the kidneys are already at the end stage). The advent of the renal
biopsy in the late 1950's raised the hope that we would learn more about
the evolution of glomerular changes. This, in fact, has not been the case
to date. Most of the reported studies have had too short a follow-up to be
significant. Striking results in the near future should not be expected,
since we know from clinical studies that the natural history of this disease
may range from 10 to 40 years.

What do we know about the diseases which might lead to end-stage
renal failure due to primary glomerular diseases? Most investigators
around the turn of the century believed that most, if not all, patients
dying in renal failure from "chronic glomerulonephritis" had followed a
slowly progressive course after an initial attack of "acute glomerulonephritis." This view has been *parroted* to the present time despite the fact
that numerous studies of post-streptococcal glomerulonephritis have
failed to find a substantial number of cases of chronic renal failure following the initial attack. In the 1970's, therefore, we are as ignorant
of the etiology of this important form of renal disease as we were when
small shrunken kidneys were first recognized at the autopsy table by
Bright.

There are a number of conditions, however, which in a relatively
short period of time following an initial insult lead to renal failure and
severely scarred kidneys. Systemic lupus erythematosus, renal artery constriction, and transplant rejection are but a few of many examples.
These, however, constitute a small portion of the total number of patients fitting into this category. The importance of understanding the
genesis of end-stage renal disease, presumed to be primarily glomerular
in origin, is that patients with this syndrome constitute the greatest majority of those requiring chronic dialysis and renal transplantation. If we,
as physicians, are to modify disease rather than treat the sequelae of
disease, it is important to understand the etiology and pathogenesis of
this condition.

Despite the fact that we know little about the etiology of this form of
end-stage renal disease, we can distinguish several broad morphologic
categories into which the majority of patients fit. As you already know
from previous sections of this chapter, the main features at this stage of
the disease will be primarily an increase in extracellular material with

distortion of the normal relationships of the glomeruli, tubules, interstitium, and vessels. The three general types are characterized as (1) proliferative and sclerosing, (2) proliferative with a lobular configuration, and (3) sclerosing, with diffuse basement membrane thickening and subepithelial deposits (so-called membranous form). (See previous section.)

End-Stage Kidney Disease Secondary to Disease of the Large Vessels (Ischemia). This form of end-stage renal disease most often accompanies a lesion in the main renal artery leading to severe *stenosis*. The affected kidney(s) becomes quite small and scarred. Histologically, the most characteristic feature is that the glomeruli appear to be relatively well preserved, whereas the tubules appear quite altered both by a decrease in size and by a change from the usual complex tubular configuration to that of a low *cuboidal* epithelium.

If the site of stenosis is in one of the major branches of the renal artery, then only a small portion of the kidney is affected; this is reflected by an irregular shrinking of the parenchyma (scarring) resulting in an irregular cortical surface. This change is seen in middle to old age, gradually increasing in severity, and is very common in diabetics.

COLLECTING AND VOIDING SYSTEM

Primary renal parenchymal lesions are presumed to be the cause of the renal failure in 75 per cent of patients with end-stage renal disease. Another 10 per cent follow congenital malformations, and 15 per cent are due to diseases of the lower urinary tract. These statistics do not give a clear indication of the clinical prevalence and morbidity associated with lower urinary tract diseases. The urinary system diseases necessitating medical care, in order of decreasing frequency, are: infection, prostatic obstruction, stones, congenital and polycystic disease, and glomerulonephritis. Therefore, lower urinary tract disease represents the bulk of clinical diseases in this system.

The function of the collecting system is to transport urine at *low pressure* and to maintain its *sterility*. Active unidirectional peristalsis takes the urine from the tip of the papilla down to the bladder in waves with a frequency of one to five times a minute. Between peristaltic waves the normal ureter collapses and is closed. The pressure in the kidney pelvis and ureter is maintained at a low level and rises only during actual peristaltic waves. At the ureterovesical junction, the oblique course of the ureter through the bladder wall forms a valve which does not allow the urine to reflux from the bladder back up into the ureter. The smooth muscle in the bladder wall and the transitional cell lining of the bladder have the function called *accommodation*, which allows the bladder to expand to accommodate large volumes of urine without increasing intravesical pressure. From the bladder, urine is expelled by a coordinated contraction of the bladder wall and relaxation of the sphincters at the bladder neck to produce complete voiding of the total bladder contents. Flow in the urethra during voiding is turbulent (has a high Reynolds number, which is proportional to diameter and velocity) and thus has a "scrubbing" action on the urethral walls, washing them free of debris and bacteria (Figure 5–49).

Obstruction. It takes relatively minor anatomic changes to interfere with the rather complex flow pattern observed in the ureter and urethra. We have used the term *obstruction to denote anything that changes the unidirectional, dynamic characteristics of flow of the urine.* As we use it, the word encompasses much more than the usual "dam in the river" type of obstruction. It includes changes in flow characteristics (e.g., from turbulent to laminar as in Figure 5–50), the formation of eddy currents in the urethra (Figure 5–51), retrograde flow of urine caused by incompetence of the urethrovesical valve, or simply the presence of a foreign surface within the urinary tract.

The presence of obstruction invites infection and calculus (stone) formation. In fact, infection, calculus, and obstruction each predispose to the others, and it is often difficult to tell which comes first.

Obstructions are divisible into two types, anatomic (or structural) and functional (e.g., neurogenic). Above the bladder, anatomic obstruction occurs frequently at the ureteropelvic segment where the pelvis narrows to join the ureter where kinks or strictures are commonly seen, or at the ureterovesical junction. Stones impacted in the ureter, blood clots, and tumors also are causes of obstruction in this segment. Anatomic obstruction occurring at the bladder neck most commonly results from benign prostatic hyperplasia (BPH) or carcinoma of the prostate, while those below the bladder neck are most commonly secondary to urethral strictures.

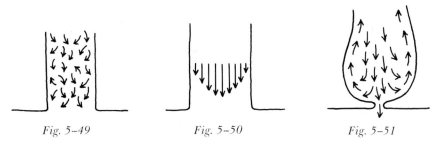

Fig. 5–49   Fig. 5–50   Fig. 5–51

Figure 5–49. Normal turbulent flow in urethra, with "scrubbing" action.

Figure 5–50. Laminar flow in urethra. Flow at center is faster than at walls; at walls, velocity approaches zero. No scrubbing action is present.

Figure 5–51. Eddy currents caused by incompetence of urethrovesical valve. Retrograde flow of urine and contaminants may occur.

Functional obstruction occurs as a result of neurologic lesions, e.g., spinal cord tumors, congenital lesions, such as meningomyelocele trauma, the neuropathy of diabetes mellitus, multiple sclerosis, or syphilis. Functional obstruction can also occur during pregnancy when the hormonally induced enlargement of the ureter and pelvis makes peristalsis less efficient (this can occur before obstruction by the gravid uterus would play a role).

The *degree* of obstruction needed to produce a clinical infection may be minimal, and it may often be difficult to demonstrate by current techniques. One of the commonest types of infection seen in females is an acute bladder infection or *cystitis*. It is known that the distal one centimeter of urethra contains bacteria. Some women with recurrent cystitis are found to have a stricture or narrowing of the urethra at the orifice or meatus (meatal stenosis). The schematic flow diagrams within a normal urethra and in one with a meatal stenosis are shown in Figures 5–49 and 5–51.

In the normal urethra it can be seen that turbulent flow has a scrubbing action on the urethral walls and washes off bacteria. Laminar flow, produced by lower flow velocities, leaves a thin layer of stationary fluid in which bacteria can survive next to the wall. With meatal stenosis, eddy currents may wash bacteria from the distal urethra back into the bladder. Thus, even relatively minor forms of obstruction may predispose to infection.

Severe obstruction below the bladder may be associated with an increased vesical pressure and cause marked hypertrophy of the muscle fibers of the bladder wall. The hypertrophied muscle bundles stand out from the wall and are visible on a cystogram, and at cystoscopy as trabeculation. As the pressure increases there is herniation of the bladder mucosa between the bundles to form *cellules*, and as these become larger and herniate through all the layers of the bladder muscle, they become *diverticula*. As the bladder enlarges it reaches its maximum capacity and loses the ability to accommodate increased volumes. The

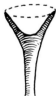
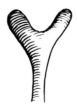
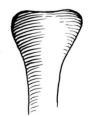

Normal cupping of calyx   Blunted   Clubbed

Figure 5-52.   Clubbing of calyx.

increased pressure and size will eventually efface the intramural portion of the ureter and make the ureterovesical valve incompetent and allow the pressure to back up to the ureter and kidneys to produce *hydroureter* and *hydronephrosis*. As the ureter becomes dilated and increases its diameter, it also increases its length and becomes tortuous and kinked. The renal pelvis enlarges, the calyces become dilated and lose the sharp *cupping* produced by the papilla projecting into the calyx, and the calyceal outline becomes club shaped (Figure 5–52).

With increased pressure in the renal pelvis, intratubular pressure increases and glomerular filtration diminishes and may stop. Renal blood flow also decreases and the renal parenchyma atrophies. The end result may be a thin-walled shell of renal parenchyma stretched over a fluid-filled pelvis. If the obstructed kidney is also infected (pyonephrosis), atrophy is markedly speeded up.

URINARY TRACT INFECTIONS (UTI)

Age, Sex, and Incidence

The normal urinary tract is sterile except near the urethral orifice. Nonetheless, infection is the most common problem of the urinary tract for which physicians are consulted. Almost every woman sometime in her life has at least one episode of acute bladder infection *(cystitis)*. The greater frequency of cystitis and bacteriuria in females as compared to males can probably be attributed to the shortness of the female urethra. From infancy until well into the second decade of life the frequency of urinary tract infections in both sexes is low. However, in the second decade, at a time when sexual intercourse begins, women manifest an abrupt increase in incidence. Urinary tract infection in males is almost restricted to those with obstructive lesions and is therefore unusual until the sixth decade of life, when the incidence increases sharply, presumably related to prostatic obstruction and its treatment.

Route of Infection

The overwhelming majority of infections are caused by enteric bacteria introduced through the urethra. The chief exception to this is the renal abscess or carbuncle, which is usually borne by the blood from another source of infection and is caused by staphylococci.

Approximately the first centimeter of the urethra is normally populated with bacteria. Above this region the urinary tract is sterile.

Bacteria introduced into the urine via the urethra are ordinarily eliminated by bladder defense mechanisms. One of these mechanisms has already been mentioned: the scrubbing of the urethral walls by the urine.

A second mechanism is the relatively complete emptying of the bladder during voiding. This can be understood by assuming that the average time needed for the bacterial population to double is $\frac{1}{2}$ hour, that the normal residual urine is 1 cc, and that the patient voids 256 cc every 3 hours (Figure 5–53).

Between voidings, the bacterial population will double every half hour and by the end of 3 hours will increase by a factor of 2^6 or 64. With voiding (from 256 cc down to 1 cc), the population will decrease by a factor of 256 with the net result that the number of bacteria is only $\frac{1}{4}$ (64/256) of what it was at the onset of the 3 hour period. If the residual is increased to only 5 cc, then the bacterial population would grow at the same rate (factor of 64) between voidings but only be decreased by a factor of 256/5 or 51, resulting in a net increase over the 3 hours. On the other hand, increasing the flow of urine and the frequency of voiding will increase the efficiency of this mechanism in preventing or ameliorating infection.

It is hypothesized that there is a third type of bladder defense mechanism having to do with the inherent antibacterial properties of the

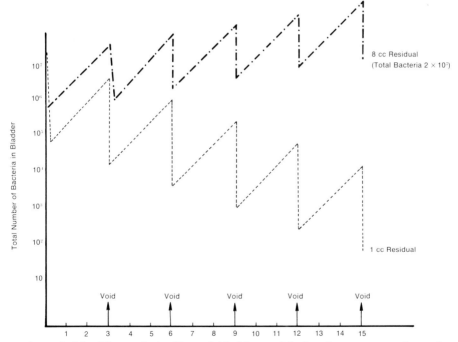

Figure 5–53. Theoretical effect of bladder residual volume on number of bacteria.

prostatic and urethral gland secretions and of the bladder mucosa itself, but little is known of this mechanism.

The retrograde flow of infected bladder urine up the ureter is the usual route bacteria take in getting to the kidney. In the normal bladder there is no retrograde flow into the ureter (reflux) during voiding. Severe obstruction, with increased bladder pressure, may make the ureterovesical valve incompetent. In the presence of infection it may also become nonfunctional, probably owing to excessive edema of the bladder wall. Extension of bacteria from the bladder to the kidney via the lymphatics has been suggested; while it is anatomically possible, it has no proven importance. The following clinical evidence supports this concept: (1) infection of the bladder urine is often demonstrable months or years before there is any sign of spread to the kidney; (2) the bacteria responsible are those found on the perineum and in prospective studies have been identified there before clinical infection occurs; (3) the occurrence of acute pyelonephritis in pregnancy is largely confined to the group of women who have bladder bacteriuria early in their course; and (4) vesico-ureteral reflux can be demonstrated radiographically in a high proportion of patients with recurrent pyelonephritis.

Clinical Manifestations of Infection

For clinical purposes infections are usually divided into those involving the lower urinary tract (cystitis, urethritis, and prostatitis) and those involving the kidney (pyelonephritis). Although many patients with urinary tract infection may be asymptomatic, when symptoms of lower urinary tract infection are present they are related to inflammation of the bladder, urethra, or prostate. *Cystitis*, although rare in men, is a very common disease in women. The typical history is of sudden onset of suprapubic discomfort, *frequency* (an urge to void every few minutes), *dysuria* (discomfort on voiding), and *urgency*, which may be severe enough to cause a precipitous, involuntary leakage of urine (urgency incontinence) if relief is not sought immediately. Even with flagrant symptoms, fever is rare with cystitis. Microscopic hematuria is common and gross hematuria is frequent. The acute attack lasts only a few days, so that symptoms and the urinalysis may clear at the end of a week even without treatment. The attack often follows sexual intercourse in women and is sometimes referred to as "honeymoon cystitis." The disease is so common in adult women that usually no search is made for an underlying obstructive process until after the third attack. In men or children, however, such an investigation is usually indicated after the first infection.

Urethritis, a common problem in men, is usually caused by a specific infection (usually gonorrhea) but may be non-bacterial (non-specific urethritis). *Gonorrhea* infections are an increasingly common problem. After venereal contact, men experience symptoms of dysuria and urethral discharge and often seek medical care early. The organisms are currently less susceptible to penicillin in many areas of the world than they were five years ago. However, adequate therapy usually eradicates the organisms. Persistent or repeated infections may result in urethral strictures and obstruction with its attendant problems. Before the advent of penicillin, gonorrhea was the commonest cause of urethral stricture. Today most strictures are iatrogenic following urethral instrumentation, but with the emergence of gonorrhea strains resistant to penicillin, the old situation may return. In women, although acute gonorrhea can cause severe pelvic pain, it sometimes produces few local symptoms; therefore medical attention may be sought relatively late. By this time, systemic infection of joints, heart valves, and tendons may have occurred. The primary areas of local infection are the uterus, the fallopian tubes, and adjacent tissue. The result is that they may become scarred and nonfunctional. Gonorrhea in women is one of the leading causes of sterility in the world. The diagnosis is made only by careful attention to the search for and culture of these fastidious organisms (*N. gonorrhoeae*), which will not grow with routine culture techniques.

The most frequent urinary tract infection in men is *prostatitis.* Here the distinction between acute and chronic forms is important. The acute stage is accompanied by fever, chills, dysuria, and sometimes difficulty passing urine or urinary retention. The acute infection involves the parenchyma of the gland around the ducts. By rectal examination, the prostate is enlarged, tense, and tender. Anything more than very gentle rectal palpation at this stage may cause septicemia or introduce bacteria into the vas deferens, producing epididymitis. Since it is a parenchymal infection, it is treated by maintaining adequate blood levels of appropriate antimicrobials.

Chronic prostatitis, in contrast, is confined mainly to the intraductal portion of the prostate and is perhaps more aptly described as a congestive prostatitis. There are usually no systemic symptoms such as chills or fever, but the patient may have poorly defined pelvic girdle or perineal aching pain. There may be frequency, but nocturia is uncommon. On rectal examination the prostate is distended and boggy. Rectal manipulation (prostatic massage) may produce prostatic fluid containing many white blood cells, in which bacteria may often not be detectable. This "infection" is within the ducts of the prostate, and since most antibiotics are not secreted into prostatic fluid they are seldom of help. The disease is significant mainly because of its frequency. Treatment is symptomatic.

As noted, *epididymitis* may complicate prostatitis and is generally an infection causing intense pain and swelling within the scrotum. (See scrotal swellings, p. 222.) It is a serious complication, as sterility may

follow a bilateral infection. Tuberculosis is a common cause of epididymitis in many areas of the world.

The characteristic clinical signs of pyelonephritis are flank pain
(produced by the edema of the kidney and stretching of the renal capsule) and a spiking fever with shaking chills. Since the infecting organisms usually ascend to the kidney, upper urinary tract infections are
often accompanied by symptoms of lower tract infection.

Laboratory Findings

The diagnosis of a urinary tract infection depends primarily upon
the demonstration of a significant number of bacteria in the urine. Since
the distal urethra normally contains bacteria, a voided specimen may
have bacteria present even though the bladder is sterile. As a practical
solution to the interpretation of bacteriuria, and in order to avoid bladder catheterization, it has been established that a urine culture obtained
from a freshly voided clean midstream specimen which contains at least
100,000 organisms per milliliter of urine represents a significant urinary
tract infection and is not likely to be due to contamination. This criterion
of 100,000 organisms per ml was selected after finding that 95 per cent
of patients with clinically diagnosed acute pyelonephritis had counts of
this magnitude or greater, whereas most obvious contaminants were in
the range of 10,000 or less per ml. Bacterial counts less than 100,000 per
ml may occur in patients with true bacteriuria. When the clean-voided
method is used, these counts can only be established as significant when
shown to be persistent and when the same species of bacteria can be
isolated.

Urinary tract infections are almost always caused by enteric organisms, with 80 per cent being due to *E. coli* in so-called uncomplicated
cases. *Proteus, Pseudomonas, Klebsiella, Enterobacter,* and various en-
terococci are more likely to be found in patients with obstruction or who
have had previous infections or instrumentation (the so-called complicated group). Many of these organisms produce urease, which can split
urea into ammonia and carbon dioxide, thus producing a characteristic
alkaline urine with an ammoniacal odor. With the production of an
alkaline urine, calcium salts frequently precipitate and increase the like-
lihood of stone formation.

Although a rare cause of urinary tract infection in this country,
tuberculosis may cause extensive destruction of the kidney, severe cystitis
with marked reduction of bladder size, or epididymitis. It warrants
special mention because it is a slowly progressive illness which may be
asymptomatic until late and because it requires special culture techniques to arrive at the diagnosis. It should be suspected when a routine
culture shows no bacterial growth in the face of symptoms and signs of
urinary tract infection.

Although it is frequently present in urinary infections, *pyuria* will not be stressed because it is often misleading when used as a single criterion of urinary tract infection, for the following reasons: (1) pus cells (neutrophils) are the hallmark of any type of inflammation, including infection, tumor, foreign bodies, and chemical or physical irritants; (2) pus cells in women may originate from the vagina during voiding.

Clinical Course

Because of the variable clinical course observed in patients with urinary infections, it has been helpful in evaluating prognosis and therapy to divide patients into four reasonably distinct categories: (1) acute uncomplicated urinary tract infections, (2) acute complicated urinary tract infections, (3) asymptomatic bacteriuria, and (4) chronic bacteriuria. The largest group of patients comprises those with acute uncomplicated urinary tract infections, and consists mainly of women who present with an initial symptomatic bout of bladder infection. *E. coli* is the usual organism, and the treatment is successful in 95 per cent of patients. Some patients who are initially thought to have uncomplicated infections are noted to have recurrences and are later found to have obstruction. This type of urinary tract infection (complicated) is particularly common in men. The outcome depends on the relief of obstruction.

Patients with asymptomatic bacteriuria, primarily women, are often discovered during the course of study for other complaints. The elderly asymptomatic men who fall in this group usually have benign prostatic hypertrophy. Obstruction is rarely found in women afflicted with this problem. Although *E. coli* is the most frequent organism found, the outcome of treatment is often poor owing to the presence of drug resistant bacteria.

The group of patients with chronic bacteriuria may have well documented, recurrent urinary tract infections, many of which are symptomatic although there may be a long asymptomatic history. Many patients have had obstructive uropathy which has failed to be corrected by surgical intervention. Organisms other than *E. coli* tend to be common in this group, and the incidence of cure of bacteriuria is less than 20 per cent with antimicrobial therapy. Chronic bacteriuria is characterized by a series of recurrent infections, which can be divided into *relapses* and *reinfections.* A relapse is defined as a recurrence with the same organism during or after therapy, while a reinfection occurs with an organism which may be of a different genus, species, or strain. The potential importance of this differentiation lies in the observations that (1) the majority of reinfections are localized in the bladder, while a significant number of relapses emanate from the kidney; and (2) many relapsing infections fail to respond to a conventional (1 to 2 week) course of antimicrobial treatment and may require more prolonged (4 to 6 week) treatment.

Acute pyelonephritis often follows or accompanies lower urinary tract infection so that the symptoms are mixed. For example, the patient commonly experiences dysuria as well as chills, fever, and costovertebral angle pain. During the infection, the urine is cloudy and contains a large number of white cells; occasionally white cell casts are noted, which are evidence that the kidney is affected. Proteinuria is minimal and azotemia is seldom a complication. Such infections seem to be episodic and self-limited when obstruction is not present. The clinical response with beginning defervescence, however, even with appropriate therapy, may take 48 hours.

Chronic pyelonephritis is a diagnosis which is difficult to establish with certainty, even histologically. Whether mild, sub-clinical infection of the kidney ever takes a chronic, indolent course cannot be stated with assurance. However, judging from the number of patients with end-stage renal failure whose disease began as acute pyelonephritis, this sequence of events is uncommon. On the basis of present knowledge, the primary rationale for vigorous treatment of urinary tract infection is the prevention of morbidity associated with infection rather than the prevention of chronic uremia. The clinical diagnosis is mainly dependent upon: (1) documented recurrent attacks of acute pyelonephritis; (2) the presence of urinary tract obstruction; (3) characteristic radiographic findings (blunting of calyces with cortical scarring overlying affected

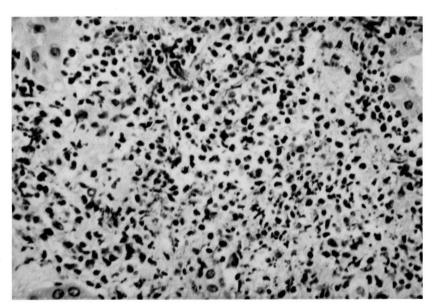

Figure 5–54 (FSB–53).   Acute pyelonephritis. The interstitium is diffusely infiltrated with acute and chronic inflammatory cells. The tubules are displaced or destroyed in these regions. Many tubules contain neutrophils.

papilla and medulla) in young patients without hypertension or other vascular disease; and (4) impaired renal function, particularly concentrating ability.

Pathology of Pyelonephritis

The macroscopic hallmarks of acute obstructive pyelonephritis are linear, yellowish streaks, radiating from the papillae to the cortex. Microscopically, the streaks are seen to be dilated tubules filled with acute inflammatory cells (Figure 5–54, FSB–53). Tubular cells may be necrotic, and the interstitium is often filled with acute inflammatory cells. If extensive damage does not occur, this lesion may heal without residual effects; however, repeated, sustained, or massive involvement leads to interstitial fibrosis and loss of nephrons. A small, shrunken kidney with large scars pitting the cortical surface appears to be the result of continued infection (Figure 5–55, FSB–54). The radiographic appearance of a chronically infected kidney reflects these abnormalities. The calyces lose their sharp margination and the ureters may become dilated (Figure 5–56, FSB–55).

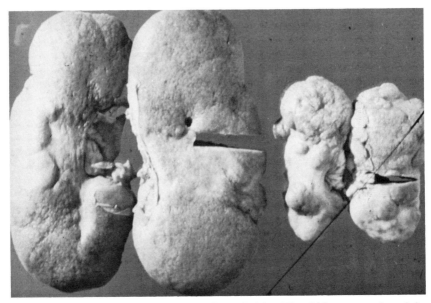

Figure 5–55 (FSB–54). Chronic pyelonephritis. The kidney on the right demonstrates the large cortical scars which result from long-standing infection secondary to chronic obstruction. The kidney on the left is from the unobstructed side.

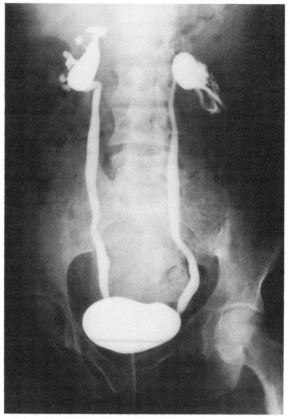

Figure 5–56 (FSB–55). Chronic pyelonephritis. A cystogram (contrast medium placed in bladder), showing bilateral vesico-ureteral reflux with small kidneys showing blunting of the calyces.

STONE FORMATION

Stones form as the result of precipitation of various salts in the collecting system. If retained, this precipitate will act as a nidus for further precipitation and thus stone growth. Therefore, anything that favors precipitation of urinary salts (increased concentration or a decrease in solubility) or the retention of the precipitate (see obstruction) will predispose to stone formation. Some precipitate may form in normal patients under appropriate conditions of diet and dehydration. This is most commonly an amorphous precipitate, but very small stones or "microliths" have been shown to form in the collecting tubules after short periods of dehydration and stress. Most stones pass out of the normal urinary tract, but if retained may act as a nidus for further deposition until a clinically significant stone is formed. A stone may serve as a focus for persistent infection or cause obstruction at one of the areas of normal narrowing of the ureter (see Chapter 2).

Prevention of stone formation is to some extent empiric (e.g., forcing fluids to dilute the urine and keep any stone salts from becoming supersaturated), but understanding of the nature and pathogenesis of stones is necessary so that specific measures can be taken for both prevention and cure. This is especially important since 50 per cent of the stones seen in clinical practice represent recurrences and might have been avoided.

A convenient division of clinical stone disease can be made into the radiopaque stones (visible on plain radiogram) and the radiolucent stones (visible only as filling defects in contrast media).

Radiopaque stones are composed of calcium and magnesium salts and comprise 95 per cent of those found in this country. Calcium oxalate stones are the most common, and are the most frequent type found in patients without a recognized associated cause (the so-called idiopathic group). Calcium phosphate and hydroxide mixtures are only slightly less common. Both types of calcium stone occur in hypercalcemic diseases, especially *hyperparathyroidism*, which accounts for about 5 per cent of clinical stones. Hypercalcemia (serum Ca > 11 mg/100 ml) should be checked for on at least three separate occasions in most calcium-stone-forming patients; if serum Ca is elevated, a detailed investigation for hyperparathyroidism should be undertaken. Hypercalciuria, such as is seen in the *immobilization of bedrest* and during *steroid therapy*, is a fairly common initiator of stones. Patients at rest after severe trauma should be encouraged to force fluids to prevent urinary tract stone formation during the inevitable bone demineralization that follows immobilization. *Renal tubular acidosis* and *infection* with urea splitting organisms also increase the incidence of calcium stones by raising the pH of the urine, which reduces the solubility of calcium salts. *Idiopathic hypercalciuria* is a syndrome seen principally in males. Serum Ca is normal but urinary calcium excretion exceeds the normal value of 300 mg/day without obvious cause.

Magnesium-ammonium-phosphate stones are the other main type of radiopaque stone and almost always are secondary to chronic infection with urea splitting organisms.

Radiolucent stones are composed of uric acid (about 5 per cent of all stones) and cystine (less than 1 per cent of all stones). Uric acid stones may occur in patients with disordered uric acid metabolism such as gout or with the tissue breakdown occurring in the treatment of lymphomas, but most are idiopathic. Because uric acid is less soluble at a low pH, patients who have consistently acid urine will form them easily. This occurs frequently in patients with persistent alkaline gastrointestinal fluid loss, such as in the chronic diarrhea of regional enteritis and ulcerative colitis, or in patients with an ileostomy. An attempt is made to alkalinize the urine in those patients who form uric acid stones in the absence of hyperuricemia. Specific protection against uric acid stones can now be provided by allopurinol, a xanthine oxidase inhibitor which reduces the oxidation of xanthine to uric acid. Using this drug, uric acid stones may slowly be dissolved over a period of months, a feat which is very difficult with calcium or magnesium calculi.

Cystine stones are diagnostic of cystinuria, a genetic disorder characterized by excessive urinary excretion of cystine, ornithine, arginine, and lysine. These stones are usually recognized by the presence of the envelope-shaped cystine crystals in the urine. As with uric acid, these crystals are insoluble in acid and the patients are often treated with alkalinization. An important advance in the treatment of cystinuria was the introduction of B-penicillamine to form mixed disulfides of cysteine and penicillamine. With the use of this agent, the excretion of free cystine can be reduced below the level associated with stone formation (about 35 mg/100 ml). It should be remembered that the presence of these stones may be but one symptom of a major metabolic disease.

Therapy for any patient with urinary stones thus depends to a considerable extent on the composition of the stone. Other important factors are the size of the stone, the presence of infection, and the severity of the symptoms. For example, a small stone causing no pain or obstruc-

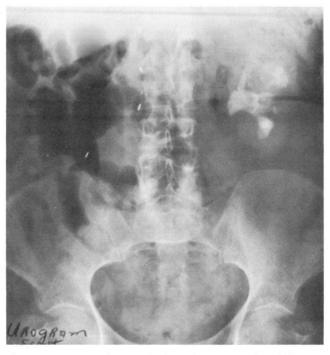

Figure 5–57 (FSB–56). Staghorn calculus: almost complete filling of the renal collecting system with radio-opaque calculus seen on an initial film of a urogram before administration of contrast media.

tion need not necessarily be removed if there is no associated urinary tract infection. An obstructing stone, or one associated with infection, should be surgically removed, both for the obstruction and because once a stone is associated with infection, it is almost impossible to clear the infection while the stone is still present. As renal stones grow they may fill the entire renal pelvis and collecting systems; because of their branched appearance they are called *staghorn* calculi (Figure 5–57, FSB–56). If left alone these staghorn calculi will usually progress to eventual destruction of the kidney. Bladder stones are less common in this country and are usually associated with bladder neck obstruction (especially benign prostatic hypertrophy).

Prophylaxis depends upon knowledge of the stone's composition and the patient's renal and lower tract function. The general principles of stone prevention are recognition and treatment of specific metabolic causes, high fluid intake to dilute the urinary solutes, treatment of infection, elimination of obstruction, and avoidance of prolonged recumbency.

TUMORS

Kidney Tumors

Since benign tumors (other than cysts) of the kidney are relatively rare, all renal masses should be considered malignant until proved

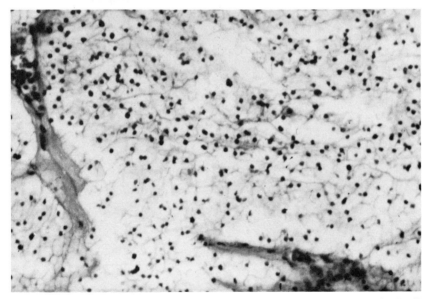

Figure 5–58 (FSB–57). Renal cell carcinoma. This tumor is composed of cells with a clear, vacuolated cytoplasm and relatively uniformly-sized nuclei.

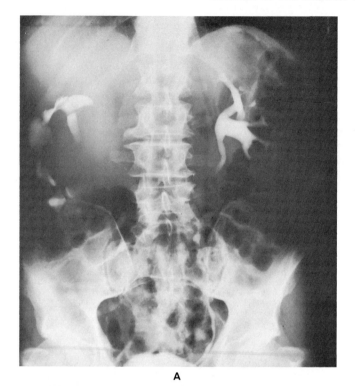

A

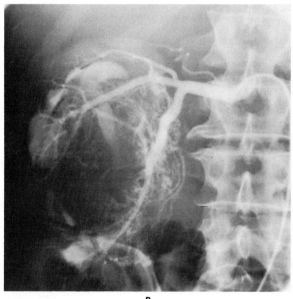

B

Figure 5-59 (FSB-58). Renal carcinoma. *A,* Excretory urogram shows filling defect in right kidney. *B,* Arterial phase blood supply with "tumor vessels" tortuous and dilated.

Figure 5-59 *continued on opposite page.*

otherwise. Histologically and clinically, the malignant renal tumors may be divided into three types: (1) renal cell carcinoma (hypernephroma or adenocarcinoma of the kidney), (2) transitional cell carcinoma of the renal pelvis, and (3) nephroblastoma (or Wilms' tumor).

Renal cell carcinoma is the most common kidney neoplasm. The incidence in men is twice that in women and increases with age. The tumor is thought to arise from renal tubular epithelium and is composed of large cells with pale vacuolated cytoplasm (Figure 5–58, FSB–57). Since these cells superficially resemble adrenal cortical tissue, an early postulate was that it arose from adrenal cell rests within the kidney. Thus, "hypernephroma" was the original name given this tumor. Renal cell carcinomas grow slowly, compressing the surrounding parenchyma.

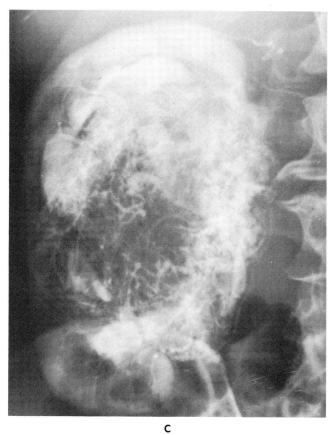

C

Figure 5–59 Continued.   C, "Tumor blush" with pooling of blood in abnormal vessels.

Spread is by direct invasion of the renal veins with dissemination through the blood stream, primarily to the lung and skeleton. The most common clinical findings in order of frequency are gross hematuria, pain, and mass. None of these signs is an early symptom. The diagnosis is usually made by an excretory urogram (Figure 5–59, FSB–58) demonstrating a space-occupying lesion distorting the normal calyceal pattern, or an angiogram showing the typical pattern of local increased vascularity.

Transitional cell carcinoma of the renal pelvis is the second most frequent kidney tumor in adults (Figure 5–60, FSB–59). Transitional cell carcinomas also occur in the ureter and bladder, where they are more common and all have the same histologic features (see below). Since the tumor is in direct contact with the urinary stream, hematuria is usually seen earlier than is the case with renal cell carcinoma. Transitional cell carcinomas of the urinary tract are commonly diagnosed by exfoliative cytology.

Wilms' tumor (nephroblastoma) is a tumor of childhood, with the peak incidence at two years of age. The tumors are composed of malignant mesenchyme which may show differentiation into primitive glomeruli and tubules (Figure 5–61, FSB–60). The tumors may be bilateral. Initially, the diagnosis may be suspected by the presence of an abdominal mass or abdominal pain and must be distinguished from neuroblastoma and hydronephrosis. The tumor is treated by a combination of surgery, chemotherapy, and radiation therapy.

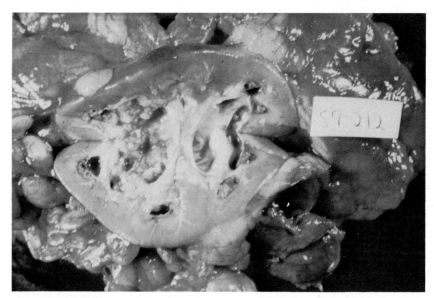

Figure 5–60 (FSB–59). Transitional carcinoma of renal pelvis. Note the papillary tumor occupying nearly half of the pelvis.

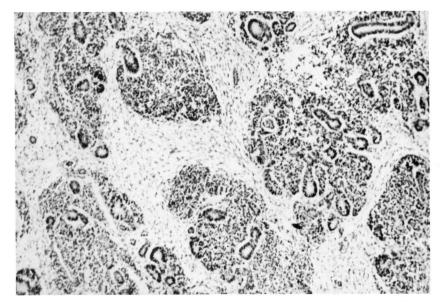

Figure 5–61 (FSB–60). Nephroblastoma. The tumor is relatively undifferentiated. Primitive tubules and glomeruli may be identified within the cellular masses.

Tumors of the Ureter and Bladder

Ninety-five per cent of all of the tumors of the ureter and bladder are *transitional cell carcinomas.* These are most frequent near the region of the trigone. Both exposure to certain aniline dyes (e.g., β-naphthylamine) and cigarette smoking have been shown to increase the incidence of these tumors. There is evidence that these tumors may be related to naturally occurring carcinogens such as some of the tryptophane metabolites excreted in the urine.

Histologically, the majority of early lesions are *papillary carcinomas* (Figure 5–62, FSB–61), which do not invade the bladder wall. As the lesions enlarge, they invade the muscle of the bladder wall and metastasize widely to local lymph nodes. Like transitional cell carcinomas of the renal pelvis, they are usually detected by the presence of painless hematuria. This symptom is common enough that gross painless hematuria should be considered bladder tumor until proved otherwise. It is important to recognize that the hematuria may be episodic and one may be misled by the apparent response to antibiotic therapy or a spontaneous clearing of the urine. Bladder tumors may often be diagnosed early (before invasion has taken place) by investigation of a single transient episode of hematuria with cystoscopy and biopsy. Early diagnosis is important because invasion of the muscle is associated with a poor prognosis (less than 15 per cent in five years if invasion is halfway through

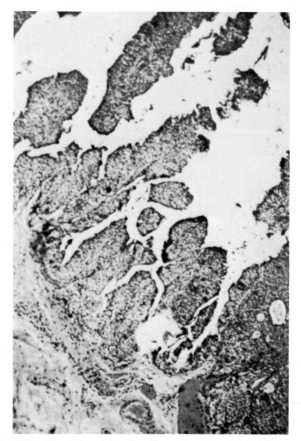

Figure 5-62 (FSB-61). Transitional cell carcinoma of bladder. Depicted is a papillary carcinoma of transitional epithelium arising in the bladder. The same histologic pattern is seen in tumors arising elsewhere in the collecting system where transitional epithelium normally resides.

muscle). Urinary cytology may be of help in making the diagnosis. The treatment is local excision for noninvasive lesions and more radical surgery (to include cystectomy) and radiation therapy for invasive tumors.

Prostatic Tumors

One-third of all males over fifty have prostatic enlargement. One-fifth of the enlargements are carcinoma, making cancer of the prostate the most common genito-urinary malignancy. Prostatic enlargement is most commonly due to "benign prostatic hyperplasia" (BPH), and BPH is the most common cause of urinary tract obstruction in the male over

60 years of age. By the age of 80 years, 75 per cent of all men have this entity. The condition is characterized by proliferation of smooth muscle, connective tissue, and prostatic acini to form a nodular mass (Figure 5–63, FSB–62). This tumor arises most commonly in the prostatic tissue *surrounding the urethra.* As the two lateral lobes enlarge, the urethral lumen is stretched and flattened and the surrounding prostatic tissue is compressed and displaced. This prostatic tumor is benign and is important only if the urinary obstruction requires operative intervention.

The symptom complex caused by BPH is called prostatism. The typical course is that of a gradual increase in nocturia, frequent, sometimes urgent voiding during the day, difficulty starting the stream with straining, and hesitancy so that it takes some time to get started. During the initial phase the bladder wall hypertrophies from working against the pressure necessary to expel the urine. This hypertrophy may be seen as thickening of the bladder wall, and trabeculation. As the process pro-

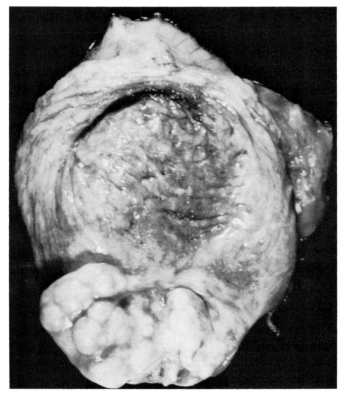

Figure 5–63 (FSB–62). Prostate hypertrophy. The urethra has been opened longitudinally and the bladder is anteriorly flattened. Note the nodular masses of prostatic tissue which bulge from the cut surface. The bladder is enlarged, has a thickened wall, and is trabeculated.

gresses, the detrusor may fail or decompensate and be unable to empty the bladder completely, leaving a *residual urine* remaining after voiding. If the bladder is allowed to rest a few minutes, the detrusor may regain its tone and empty the bladder with a second effort. This type of double or triple voiding is known as *intermittency*. It can be seen that if a significant residual volume is present, the *effective bladder capacity* is reduced (i.e., if bladder capacity is 300 cc and 200 cc of residual urine exists, the effective capacity is only 100 cc), and voiding will be more frequent. In some cases the first symptom may be an acute episode of retention, with the patient unable to void at all.

Occasionally an individual with a high residual urine volume will remain asymptomatic while his bladder gradually distends to enormous size and the ureter and pelvis become dilated. He may present with signs of uremia, weakness, nausea, vomiting, weight loss, straw-colored skin, and a large abdominal mass which disappears after insertion of the urethral catheter and decompression of the bladder. This is called silent prostatism.

As mentioned previously, in prostatic hyperplasia the periurethral glands enlarge. When this happens, one can distinguish different areas of the gland, and these are called the *lobes* of the prostate. The most common areas of enlargement are on either side of the urethra and are called the lateral lobes. Lateral lobe enlargement broadens the gland, and the enlargement can be palpable on rectal examination. Flattening of the urethra in the transverse diameter and splaying in the anteroposterior diameter can be demonstrated on a urethrogram. Median lobe enlargement occurs at the posterior bladder neck, and usually the adenoma bulges into the bladder. It obstructs with a ball valve effect at the bladder neck. Because of its position it is not palpable as an enlargement on rectal examination.

These "lobes" of adenomatous hyperplasia are surrounded by an area of compressed normal prostatic tissue called the surgical capsule. Treatment of BPH is surgical and consists of removal of the adenomatous tissue, leaving the surgical capsule intact.

Carcinoma of the Prostate

Adenocarcinoma of the prostate is one of the more common malignancies in men over the age of fifty, accounting for almost 10 per cent of male cancer deaths in the U. S. (estimated at 17,600 for 1972). The incidence increases with age, and histological evidence of carcinoma can be found in more than 25 per cent of men over the age of eighty years. While men under the age of sixty usually have rapidly progressive disease, older men are often asymptomatic because the tumor is slowly growing and may remain localized for some time.

Prostatic cancer is usually an adenocarcinoma arising from the glandular epithelium (Figure 5–64, FSB–63). Fortunately, most prostatic carcinomas occur in the posterior lobe. The diagnosis can thus be picked up early on rectal examination by the finding of a hard nodule or, more frequently, a localized change in consistency of the prostate. Definitive diagnosis can be made by needle biopsy obtained through the perineum or the rectum. The acinar cells of the prostate produce large quantities of acid phosphatase, which normally is excreted in the urine. If there is metastatic disease or capsular invasion, acid phosphatase may escape

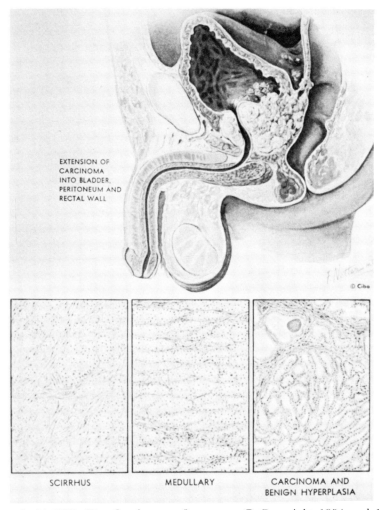

EXTENSION OF CARCINOMA INTO BLADDER, PERITONEUM AND RECTAL WALL

© Ciba

SCIRRHUS   MEDULLARY   CARCINOMA AND BENIGN HYPERPLASIA

Figure 5–64 (FSB–63). Carcinoma of prostate. © Copyright 1954 and 1965 CIBA Pharmaceutical Company, division of CIBA-GEIGY Corporation. Reproduced, with permission, from THE CIBA COLLECTION OF MEDICAL ILLUSTRATIONS by Frank H. Netter, M.D. All rights reserved.

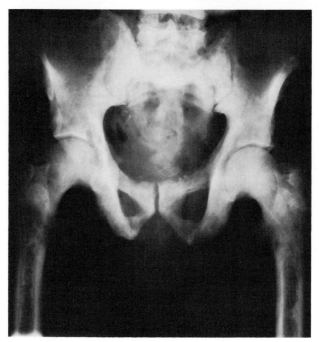

Figure 5–65 (FSB–64). Carcinoma of prostate: bony metastases.

into the blood stream. Resulting elevated serum levels help establish the diagnosis of extra-capsular prostatic carcinoma.

Carcinoma of the prostate spreads locally into the prostatic capsule and seminal vesicle by direct invasion. In the early part of its course it spreads into the perineural lymphatics and pelvic lymph nodes. Later it spreads by venous channels into the vertebral system, and often the first symptom is pain caused by metastatic disease in the spine (Figure 5–65, FSB–64).

Treatment of the early localized lesion may be radical surgery, but this is applicable in only about 3 per cent of the cases since most of the tumors have spread beyond the capsule by the time the diagnosis is made. Androgen suppression by either orchiectomy or administration of estrogens may shrink these tumors, since they tend to be hormonally dependent. Radiation therapy to the primary tumor and to symptomatic metastases has also been used.

Scrotal Masses

Most masses in the scrotum which are outside the testes are benign, while all masses in the testicles are *malignant*. Nontesticular tumors are uncommon (even though it is the most common malignant tumor of the male in the 25 to 35 year age group) but may be fatal since metastases occur early.

The testes form as retroperitoneal organs which descend into the scrotum at the time of birth (Figure 5–66, FSB–65). An elongated pouch of peritoneum (processus vaginalis) accompanies the testis into the scrotum. This pouch becomes entirely obliterated except for the distal

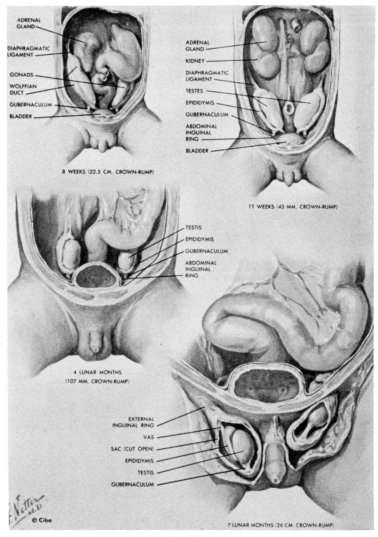

portion, which surrounds the testis to become the tunica vaginalis. If the processus vaginalis remains open, abdominal contents may descend into the inguinal canal and scrotum to form an inguinal hernia. Hernias are generally non-tender and reduce (return to normal position) when the patient lies down, but may be painful if incarcerated (impacted into the inguinal canal so that reduction into the peritoneal cavity is impossible), or *strangulated* (pinched to cause obstruction).

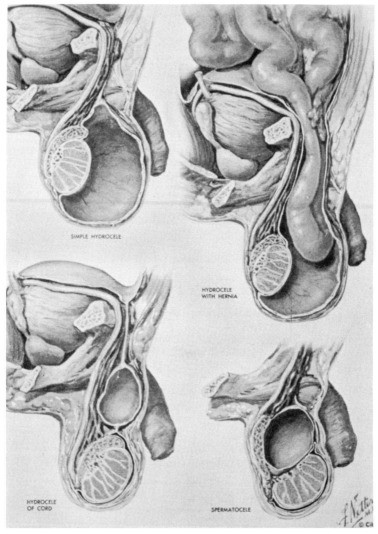

Figure 5–67 (FSB–66). Hydrocele and spermatocele. © Copyright 1954 and 1965 CIBA Pharmaceutical Company, division of CIBA-GEIGY Corporation. Reproduced, with permission, from THE CIBA COLLECTION OF MEDICAL ILLUSTRATIONS by Frank H. Netter, M.D. All rights reserved.

Distension of the tunica vaginalis by straw-colored fluid is called a *hydrocele* (Figure 5–67, FSB–66). The testis is entirely inside the fluid and, if the hydrocele is tense, the testis cannot be palpated. Hydroceles can usually be transilluminated. They are very common in infants, but most of them disappear spontaneously. In the adult they are removed only if large enough to be symptomatic.

The *spermatocele* is a small, non-tender cystic enlargement occurring in the rete testis (between the upper pole of the testis and the epididy-

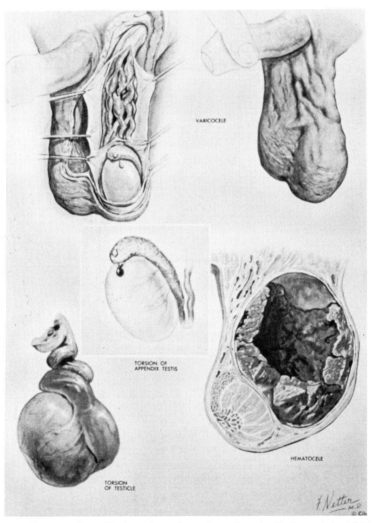

Figure 5–68 (FSB–67). Varicocele and torsion of testis. © Copyright 1954 and 1965 CIBA Pharmaceutical Company, division of CIBA-GEIGY Corporation. Reproduced, with permission, from THE CIBA COLLECTION OF MEDICAL ILLUSTRATIONS by Frank H. Netter, M.D. All rights reserved.

mis). A spermatocele can usually be palpated as a mass distinct from the testis and is sometimes mistaken for a third testis. (This is known as the "pawn shop sign.") The spermatocele is filled with fluid, which is either gray or opalescent white, from the seminiferous tubules. Like the hydrocele, a spermatocele is removed only if it produces symptoms or a problem in diagnosis.

A *varicocele* is a plexus (pampiniform plexus) of dilated veins lying just above the testis (Figure 5–68, FSB–67). On physical examination, a varicocele feels like a "bag of worms." Since the veins are filled with blood, in contrast to hydroceles, they do not transilluminate. They may be associated with a dull, dragging discomfort, but more often are asymptomatic. The varicocele is common on the left and rare on the right, because of the difference in venous drainage.

The epididymis is palpable as a soft tubular structure on the posterior aspect of the testis. The vas deferens courses from the inferior pole of the epididymis and joins the main portion of the spermatic cord in the upper scrotum. *Epididymitis* may be localized early in its evolution, but often goes unnoticed until the edema surrounding the epididymis is massive enough to make it appear as though the whole testis were swollen. In the diagnosis of epididymitis, a history of urinary tract infection or instrumentation is common. Onset is usually within a period of an hour, the urine usually contains WBC's, and an associated prostatitis is common.

Epididymitis must be distinguished from *torsion of the spermatic cord* (Figure 5–68), which is a urological emergency. If a torsion is not reduced (untwisted) within six hours, a non-viable testis results. Torsion of the testis is characterized by immediate acute onset, severe pain, retracted testis, and abnormal location of epididymis. Most cases occur below 18 years of age, while epididymitis rarely does. The defect allowing torsion is an abnormal attachment of the testis to the scrotal wall. It is often bilateral.

Tumors of the Testis

Tumors of the testis are relatively uncommon, but their peak incidence is in the young male (15 to 35 years), making them among the common tumors in this age group. They usually present as a firm, nontender mass, often found after a blow to the testis has called attention to the area. Unfortunately, they are aggressive and metastasize early, usually first via lymphatics (to the retroperitoneal lymph nodes), and later via the veins (to the lung).

Classification of the tumors of the testis has been difficult, and several systems of nomenclature have been proposed. Most tumors are of germinal cell origin and are of the teratoma group, although only

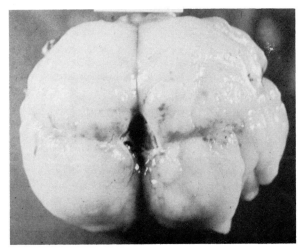

Figure 5–69 (FSB–68). Seminoma. This tumor is composed of a uniform mass of tissue which has a white color.

rarely are they well enough differentiated to be considered benign. Usually they are a mixture of histological cell types and, for obvious clinical reasons, the name applied is that of the cell type with the worst prognosis.

At one end of the prognostic scale are the seminomas (20 to 40 per cent of the testis tumors) (Figure 5–69, FSB–68; Figure 5–70, FSB–69).

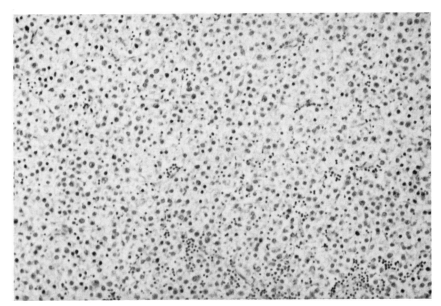

Figure 5–70 (FSB–69). Microscopically, the seminoma is composed of relatively large cells with vacuolated cytoplasm and pleomorphic nuclei. Scattered throughout are aggregations of small leukocytes.

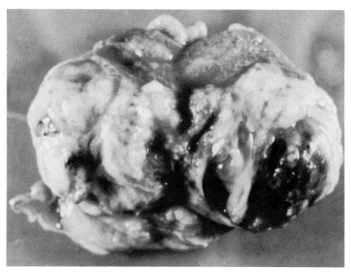

Figure 5-71 (FSB-70). Teratoma. The tumor is composed of several types of malignant tissues. It is rapidly growing and hemorrhagic.

The seminomas have a good prognosis, not because of normal untreated behavior but because they are highly radio-sensitive.

At the other end of the scale are teratomas (Figure 5-71, FSB-70), teratocarcinomas, or embryonal cell carcinomas, and choriocarcinomas, which are relatively insensitive to radiation and have a worse prognosis.

About 10 per cent of testicular tumors produce chorionic gonadotrophin which is excreted in the urine. A positive urine test, found in a patient who seems to have a seminoma or teratoma, indicates that the tumor has carcinomatous elements in it. Persistance of an elevated chorionic gonadotrophin after removal of the testis suggests the presence of functioning metastases.

Chapter 6

A CLINICAL
APPROACH TO
DISEASES OF THE
URINARY SYSTEM

When the patient dies the kidneys may go to the pathologist, but while he lives the urine is ours. It can provide us day by day, month by month, and year by year with a serial story of the major events going on within the kidney.

THOMAS ADDIS (1881–1949)

It is axiomatic that patients come to a physician for help with medical problems. In the previous chapters the anatomy, physiology, and diseases of the urinary system were discussed. This was done by starting with the normal and then discussing pathological entities and the effects which they have upon the entire body. Unfortunately, to use this information in a clinical setting it must be turned around and looked at from the point of view of the symptoms with which the patient presents. Such symptoms are not always easily interpreted by the patient or physician, but a proper solution is always dependent upon the amount and accuracy of the data available and its correct interpretation. Symptoms related to disorders of the urinary system are frequently vague and nonspecific. Diagnosis of disease in the urinary system depends in great measure on the classical determinants of any clinical disorder; that is, the historic or subjective data base obtained from patient observations, and the objective data base obtained by the physician through physical examination and laboratory tests. This chapter will describe: (1) data that suggest urinary system disease; (2) clinical data analysis; and (3) the treatment of patients with end-stage renal failure.

THE SUBJECTIVE DATA BASE

Changes in Micturition. The healthy person voids about every 4 to 6 hours, excretes the majority of his urine during the daytime, and

229

does not normally void urine at night. Frequent micturition (*frequency*), when not associated with an increase in urine volume, is a symptom of decreased *effective* bladder capacity often related to disorders of the lower urinary tract such as infection or obstruction. Typically, urine flow decreases at night, so that nocturnal voidings (*nocturia*) is an abnormal symptom but is not specific; it is usually related to the same causes of diurnal frequency noted previously. Occasionally, nocturia may be an early symptom of cardiac and hepatic failure without evidence of intrinsic urinary system disease. In this case, the nocturia is related to a mild diuresis at night associated with the assumption of a prone position.

Painful urination (*dysuria*) suggests an irritative or inflammatory process in the bladder neck or urethra. Frequently, it is associated with bacterial infection of the urinary tract. In the absence of bacterial infection, a careful evaluation of the bladder and urethra should be made if the symptoms persist.

Change in Urinary Output.   The normal daily urinary output in adults varies between 700 and 2000 ml. Renal disease producing functional impairment may be associated with *polyuria* (greater than 2500 ml daily) or *oliguria* (less than 500 ml daily). In progressive renal insufficiency, mild polyuria (3 to 4 liters daily) is a common symptom of failing renal function. It is little influenced by fluid restriction, and is the result of a concentrating defect and a relative osmotic diuresis in the remaining functional nephrons. Oliguria occurs in many acute conditions due to decreased renal perfusion (pre-renal factors), ureteral or bladder outlet obstruction (post-renal factors), or primary renal disease.

The most extreme form of oliguria is *anuria* (less than 100 ml daily), which is inevitably associated with uremia. It may be a manifestation of acute renal failure or the end stage of chronic progressive renal insufficiency. Anuria may also be due to total urinary obstruction, so that urologic evaluation should be considered.

Change in Urine Color.   Depending on the degree of solute concentration, urine may vary from clear when dilute, to a deep yellow color when maximally concentrated due to the presence of urobilin. In the absence of drug or food pigment excretion, an abnormal discoloration of urine is an indication of clinical disease (hematuria, hemoglobinuria, myoglobinuria, pyuria, porphyria, or melanoma). A cloudy urine frequently indicates pyuria due to a urinary tract infection, but a similar cloudiness is often caused by precipitated amorphous phosphate salts if the urine is alkaline. Microscopy of the urinary sediment will answer this question.

The presence of blood in the urine may produce a red to brown discoloration, depending on the amount present and the acidity of the urine. Lesser degrees of hematuria may cause no discoloration and may only be detected by microscopic determination. When hematuria is noted, the presence or absence of pain related to the urinary system is important. Hematuria without pain is usually due to renal, vesical, or prostatic disease, whereas painful hematuria is most often associated with ureteral or urethral obstruction from stones, blood clots, or tumor.

Pain. The pain related to renal disease is usually situated in the flank or back between the 12th rib and the iliac crest, with occasional radiation to the epigastrium. Stretching of the pain-sensitive renal capsule is the probable cause of discomfort and may occur in any condition producing parenchymatous swelling, such as acute glomerulonephritis, acute pyelonephritis, nephrolithiasis, polycystic disease, and occasionally renal carcinoma. There is often marked tenderness over the kidney in the angle formed by the 12th rib and the lumbar spine.

Irritation of the renal pelvis or ureter causes pain in the flank and hypochondrium, with radiation into the ipsilateral iliac fossa and often into the upper thigh, testicle, or labium. The pain is intermittent, but does not completely remit between waves of colic.

Edema. Edema is a common manifestation of nephropathy. There is no single type of edema produced only by renal disease. The complex mechanisms which maintain a constant extracellular volume in health may be upset in many ways by heart, liver or kidney disease. Whatever the primary cause, edema always represents excessive water and sodium salts in the extracellular space due to abnormal reabsorption in both the proximal and distal nephron. In the initial stages, the retention of sodium and water is evident only by an increase in weight, but later edema becomes overt. Edema associated with renal disease is often first noticeable as facial puffiness rather than ankle swelling, but these characteristics are neither essential nor specific. If fluid retention continues, generalized edema (*anasarca*) with fluid transudates (*effusions*) in the pleural and peritoneal cavities may be seen. Such a condition is most often associated with the nephrotic syndrome (Chapter 5).

Failure to Thrive. Most patients with progressive decompensation of the urinary system are asymptomatic. However, when sufficient renal function is lost (GFR <10% of normal), disturbances of multiple organ systems occur, producing symptoms ascribable to uremia. Weight loss, weakness, fatigue, dyspnea, anorexia, nausea and vomiting, itching, failure to grow, tetany, peripheral neuropathy, and convulsions are the usual signs and symptoms. They are apparently related to retention of various metabolic products, and most of them can be ameliorated or reversed by adequate dialysis or renal transplantation and good nutrition.

Past Medical History. A previous history of hypertension, systemic disease (diabetes mellitus, SLE, etc.), renal disease, trauma to the urinary system, stones, or prior urinary system surgery is of great importance. In addition, a family history of renal disease in an adult may suggest polycystic disease or, if associated with ear and eye disorders, may indicate hereditary nephritis. A history of recent infectious diseases involving the skin, respiratory tract, or endocardium is helpful in evaluating possible causes of glomerulonephritis.

THE OBJECTIVE DATA BASE

Patient Examination. *Hypertension* is commonly associated with renal disease (vascular obstruction, glomerulonephritis), especially in childhood. However, no more than 10 per cent or so of adult hypertensive patients have renovascular causes. Progressive renal failure is associated with hypertension in most patients only when the ECV is expanded, and the condition can be controlled by sodium restriction. The relationship between renal disease and hypertension is complex and poorly understood despite much clinical and experimental study.

The *skin* may show pallor, suggesting anemia, or a yellowish brown pigment due to a retention of urochromes; excoriations may be present, suggesting pruritus; and infections, either carbuncles or cellulitis, may be present. Occasionally, skin lesions from vasculitis or endocarditis may be present, thus suggesting a possible cause of renal disease. The *optic fundi* are useful in an evaluation of vascular disease, and should also be examined for the presence of hemorrhages, exudates, and papilledema. The *mouth* may reveal stomatitis or an odor of urine, while a look at the *face*, *abdomen*, or *extremities* may reveal edema. Palpation of enlarged *kidneys*, *bladder* or *prostate* is an important clue in the diagnosis of urinary system disease.

Laboratory Data. The patient with chronic renal insufficiency typically develops a hypoproliferative *anemia*. An elevated or progressively increasing BUN and creatinine indicate a decreased glomerular filtration rate. The finding of a depressed serum bicarbonate may indicate the presence of a metabolic acidosis due to renal insufficiency or a tubular defect. An elevated serum calcium or globulin may point toward other causes of renal dysfunction.

An important test of intrinsic urinary system disease is the *urinalysis.* The usual urine examination involves a qualitative evaluation of certain chemical constituents and microscopic examination of the sediment. The customary technique of urinalysis has been greatly simplified in recent years by the development of a simple dipstick. These dipsticks are clear plastic strips to which are affixed pieces of cellulose material impregnated with various reagents. They are designed to test urine specimens for the presence of protein, glucose, ketones, bilirubin, and blood and to indicate the urinary pH. Additionally, it is common to measure the solute concentration of urine by either refractometry or osmometry. A brief comment will be made regarding each of these urine tests.

Proteinuria. The dipstick technique is sensitive to as little as 5 to 20 mg of albumin per 100 ml of urine, but is less sensitive to globulins, Bence-Jones protein, and mucoproteins. This difference in sensitivity is of little chemical significance because in most renal diseases albumin predominates, although the urine may also contain other proteins. Persistent proteinuria is due to renal disease, but transient proteinuria may be associated with disease in other organ systems such as congestive heart failure. Although qualitative testing is adequate to ferret out abnormalities, quantitative measurements of protein excretion are useful in suggesting certain types of renal disease and in following the clinical progress of patients. Quantitative assessment of the proteinuria is usually done by collecting urine for 24 hours and measuring the total protein content. As measured by this technique, the normal subject excretes less than 150 mg of protein daily. An alternate technique is to assess the amount of protein (mg/100 ml) present in relation to the creatinine content (mg/100 ml) of a random sample of urine. In a normal patient, the protein/creatinine ratio is less than 0.1. Heavy proteinuria (> 2 g/m^2/day or a protein/creatinine ratio >2) is usually found in patients with glomerular disease producing the nephrotic syndrome. Smaller amounts of proteinuria may be seen with other types of nephropathy.

Glycosuria. This is commonly detected by one of two methods: (1) a dipstick which is impregnated with glucose oxidase, or (2) the reduction of dilute alkaline copper solution (Benedict's reagent or Clinitest tablets). The latter test is less sensitive, and responds to other reducing substances such as lactose, levulose, pentose, galactose, and ascorbic acid. The dipstick test is both specific and very sensitive, with a response to as little glucose as 100 mg/100 ml of urine.

Possible causes of glycosuria include the following:

1. Hyperglycemia with normal renal glucose threshold.
   a. Endocrinopathies: diabetes mellitus, glucocorticoidism, pheochromocytoma, thyrotoxicosis.
   b. Alimentary hyperglycemia due to excessive intestinal absorption.
   c. Rapid glucose infusions.
2. Normoglycemia with reduced renal glucose threshold.
   a. Proximal tubular dysfunction—may be an isolated defect or part of a more generalized defect (Fanconi's syndrome).

Ketonuria. This is diagnosed by the dipstick which is impregnated with sodium nitroprusside. This reagent detects small amounts of acetoacetic acid, but is less sensitive to acetone and does not react with beta-hydroxybutyric acid. Ketonuria is common in two conditions:

1. Starvation—ketosis is mild, and ketones are found in plasma in low concentrations if at all detectable.
2. Uncontrolled diabetes mellitus—ketosis and acidosis may be profound and ketones are easily detected in the plasma.

Hematuria. This condition is best appreciated by microscopic examination. However, a dipstick impregnated with a buffered mixture of organic peroxide and orthotolidine is sensitive to free hemoglobin and myoglobin. A positive dipstick test and the absence of red blood cells on microscopic examination suggest the presence of free hemoglobin or myoglobin in the urine.

Other Chemical Tests.   There are many other examinations to which urine can be subjected for special purposes. These include the following:

1. Bilirubin — positive in patients with jaundice who have at least some conjugated bilirubin.
2. Urobilinogen — positive in patients who don't have total biliary obstruction and are secreting bile into their gut.
3. Amino acids — qualitative tests are needed to distinguish generalized aminoaciduria seen in proximal tubular defects (Fanconi's syndrome) from that seen in patients with specific enzyme deficient states such as cystinuria, Hartnup's disease, etc.
4. Steroids — useful in the diagnosis of endocrine abnormalities.
5. Xylose — used to detect intestinal malabsorption by measuring the amount of xylose excreted after a standard oral dose.

Urine pH.   The pH is measured by a dipstick which is impregnated with various dyes which respond to hydrogen ion in the pH range of 5 to 9. There is no particular reason for its routine measurement, as it will neither identify nor exclude patients with urinary system disease. However, it is often useful in identifying various crystals which may be present in urine on microscopy. Specific pH testing is critical in the diagnosis of the "distal" type of renal tubular acidosis (Chapter 4). In this case, a metabolic acidosis, *if not already present*, is produced by oral loading with ammonium chloride, and the renal response is noted by measuring titratable acid and ammonium excretion and the urine pH with a hydrogen-ion-sensitive glass electrode. Inability to lower urine pH below 5.5 and to increase titratable acid or ammonium to appropriate levels following the development of systemic acidosis is considered abnormal. Patients with advanced renal failure can usually vary urinary pH in a relatively normal manner, although the quantitative capacity to excrete titratable acid and ammonium is reduced.

Renal Concentrating Capacity.   This test is sensitive to early renal dysfunction and correlates well with histologic changes in the tubulo-interstitial area. The concentration of solutes in urine is most often measured by specific gravity, refractive index or osmolality. Although osmolality measurement by freezing point determination is the ideal way to evaluate renal concentrating and diluting capacity, refractometry and specific gravity are currently the most commonly used measurements. The latter two measurements require correction for abnormal amounts of urine protein and glucose. The relationship of specific gravity to osmolality is illustrated in Figure 6–1. It is clear that the relationship is not linear and that at any given osmolality, a wide variation in the specific gravity may be seen. This is particularly true when substances such as glucose or the contrast chemicals used in urography are present.

The routine measurement of urine osmolality on random urine samples is not helpful except when the urine osmolality is >700

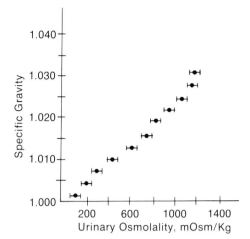

Figure 6-1. The correlation between specific gravity and urinary osmolality.

mOsm/L (specific gravity >1.020). The capacity to concentrate to this degree indicates reasonably good renal function, but a value below this may be entirely normal if the patient has suppressed his level of antidiuretic hormone by fluid ingestion or is undergoing an osmotic diuresis. Renal concentrating capacity is best tested by two procedures: (1) water deprivation for a period of 18 to 24 hours, and (2) the response to exogenous vasopressin administration. A response to vasopressin and a lack of response to water deprivation suggests an endogenous deficiency of ADH. A lack of response to either water deprivation or exogenous vasopressin suggests an intrinsic renal concentrating defect which may be due to one or more of the following:

1. Functional tubular impairment
   a. Congenital
      (1) Nephrogenic diabetes insipidus
      (2) Fanconi's syndrome
   b. Acquired
      (1) Osmotic diuresis
      (2) Certain diuretics (furosemide, ethacrynic acid)
      (3) Potassium deficiency
      (4) Hypercalcemia
2. Tubulointerstitial disease
   a. Sickle cell disease
   b. Toxic nephritis (e.g., analgesics, methacillin, sulfa)
   c. Pyelonephritis
   d. Any end-stage renal disease (e.g., CGN, RPGN)

The Urinary Sediment Examination.   In health, the urine contains a small number of cells and other formed elements from the whole length of the urinary system. With renal parenchymal disease, the urine usually contains increased numbers of cells and casts which may provide information useful for diagnosis. In the case of urinary tract infections, fractionation of a voided urine sample may give useful information as to the site of inflammation.

Examination of the urinary sediment should be done with a well-mixed, fresh urine sample. If examination is delayed, the urine should be stored in a refrigerator. Urine should be collected in clean containers, avoiding obvious sources of contamination such as vaginal discharge. If the lesion is thought to be in the lower urinary tract in men, three successive specimens should be collected during voiding. The initial 5 ml of urine would represent urethral cells, the mid-volume would represent bladder urine, and the final 5 to 10 ml of urine at the end of micturition would represent the prostatic and bladder neck cytology.

There are two ways of separating the particulate matter in urine from the urine water. Forcing urine through a filter of appropriate pore size is a way of rapidly accomplishing this task, but requires special facilities to stain and prepare the filter and sediment for microscopic examination. It does, however, offer the advantage of a permanent record of the urinary system cytology. The more common technique is to centrifuge the urine specimen and inspect the sediment "button" at the bottom of the tube. It is most helpful to place the sediment button in a hemocytometer chamber, although an ordinary glass slide and cover slip will suffice. A portion of the button may be stained, if desired, to exaggerate the different types of cells present. The Prescott-Brodie stain is particularly useful in distinguishing leukocytes from epithelial cells. Correct use of the microscope is of great importance; with the ordinary equipment, one should use subdued light by lowering the condensor and closing the diaphragm. Best results are obtained with examination first under low power, and later at higher magnifications to identify abnormalities when seen. Phase microscopy is very helpful when available.

Table 6-1.   Classification of Urinary Formed Elements.

1. Cells from blood:	
a. Erythrocytes	c. Lymphocytes
b. Leukocytes	d. Plasma cells, etc.
2. Cells from urinary system:	
a. Renal: tubular cells (with or without fat)	
b. Lower tract: transitional and squamous cells, sperm	
3. Foreign cells:	
a. Bacteria	c. Parasites
b. Fungi	d. Neoplastic
4. Crystals:	
a. Oxalate	c. Urates
b. Phosphates	d. Drugs, etc.

Interpretation of the Urinary Sediment.   As demonstrated in Table 6–1, there is marked variability of the formed elements seen in the urinary sediment. It is clear that cells are desquamated into urine from all parts of the urinary system, and uncatheterized samples from women always contain cells from the genital tract as well. It is uncommon to observe more than one leukocyte, erythrocyte, or epithelial cell per high power field in the normal male, or more than four leukocytes per high field in the normal woman. An increased number of cells should alert the physician to disease in the urinary system. Excessive numbers of red cells may indicate infection, tumor, stones, or inflammation. Excessive leukocytes may indicate infection or other inflammatory diseases. The finding of bacteria in a centrifuged urinary sediment is not necessarily evidence of a significant urinary tract infection. However, the finding of bacteria in an uncentrifuged fresh urine sample is common, with urine cultures of greater than 10^5 organisms/ml of voided urine.

The element in urine sediment examination of greatest importance in distinguishing primary renal disease from diseases of the lower tract is the finding of casts. Casts are cylindrical masses of mucoprotein in which cellular elements, protein, or fat droplets may be entrapped. The possible types of casts and the diseases with which they are associated are noted in Table 6–2.

Red blood cell casts are of great significance because they are virtually pathognomonic of glomerulonephritis when present in large numbers. It has been stated that the white cell cast is pathognomonic of pyelonephritis, but in actuality the finding of such casts is only indicative of tubulointerstitial inflammation, and they are commonly seen in certain stages of proliferative glomerulonephritis and forms of interstitial nephritis which may or may not be related to bacterial infection.

The type of cast seen is often useful in suggesting the *cause* and *severity* of renal involvement. In patients with far advanced renal failure, waxy and broad casts containing different inclusions are often seen. The width of the cast excreted in the urine is presumably a model of the tubular area from which it was excreted, and it is thus likely that the broad casts represent cast formations in the collecting duct area, a finding which suggests diffuse, widespread nephron involvement.

Diagnosis of Bacterial Infections of the Urinary System.   Bacteria found in voided urine may enter as contaminants in collection vessels, from periurethral tissues, from the urethra itself, from gross fecal or vaginal contamination, or from organisms actually multiplying in the urine. The concept of "significant bacteriuria" was introduced to distinguish among these possibilities. This can be accomplished by knowledge of the site and manner in which the urine is collected from the patient and the number of organisms present in the sample. Aseptic methods of collection of urine from the renal pelvis, ureter, or bladder permit the diagnosis of significant bacteriuria regardless of the number of orga-

Table 6–2. Classification of Urinary Casts.

---

1. Plain Casts
   a. Hyaline cast—Mucoprotein matrix secreted by tubular cells, with a refractive index close to that of water. Seen best in subdued light.
      1. Without renal disease: reduced renal blood flow, as with exercise or heart failure.
      2. With renal disease: non-specific but usually those that involve the glomeruli.
   b. Waxy cast—Casts which have remained stagnant in tubules long enough to become completely homogenized. Matrix consists of serum proteins. Form in distal nephron, and thus are larger than hyaline cast.
      1. Advanced renal failure.

2. Casts with Inclusions
   a. Red cell cast—Hyaline cast whose matrix is variably filled with red cells. Appears red-orange in both unstained and stained sediments because of the color of the red cells.
      1. Proliferative glomerulonephritis (always).
      2. Cortical necrosis (usually).
      3. Acute tubular injury (occasionally).
   b. Epithelial cell casts—Cast composed entirely of tubular epithelial cells without much protein matrix.
      1. Acute tubular injury.
      2. Glomerulonephritis.
      3. Nephrotic syndrome.
   c. Pus cast—Hyaline cast containing one or more leukocytes.
      1. Proliferative glomerulonephritis.
      2. Pyelonephritis or interstitial nephritis.
   d. Mixed cast—Hyaline cast containing red cells, tubular epithelial cells, and/or leukocytes.
      1. Proliferative glomerulonephritis.
   e. Fatty cast—Hyaline cast containing fat droplets in epithelial cells.
      1. Nephrotic syndrome.
   f. Other inclusions—Crystals, bacteria.

3. Pseudo-casts—Clumped urates, leukocytes, bacteria, mucus, and artifacts. Important to distinguish from true casts.

---

nisms found, provided that the specimen is not contaminated prior to culture. The criterion of 100,000 or more organisms per milliliter of urine for diagnosis of significant bacteriuria is primarily of diagnostic significance when the clean-voided method is employed to collect specimens.

The question is often asked, "When should a patient be catheterized for collection of urine for culture?" Catheterization (either urethral or suprapubic) is sometimes necessary in patients who are suspected of being obstructed, who cannot void, or who are too ill or too weak to permit collection of a clean-voided specimen. Catheter specimens may

Table 6-3.   Clinical Tests of Renal Function.

FUNCTION	SPECIFIC TEST	CLINICAL TEST
Glomerular filtration	Inulin clearance ^{125}I-Iothalamate clearance	Creatinine clearance Plasma creatinine Plasma urea (BUN)
Renal plasma flow	PAH clearance	PSP excretion
Proximal tubular	Tm glucose (reabsorption) Tm PAH (secretion)	Plasma phosphate, urate PSP excretion Urinary amino acids
Distal tubular	Max. U/P osmolality Acidifying capacity: pH, TA, NH_4^+	Maximal urinary osmolality Acid load test

frequently be much lower in bacterial content than voided samples and still indicate infection.

Measurement of Renal Function. Various tests have been suggested to measure the physiological integrity of the kidney in health and disease. In general, these can be divided into classes according to measurement of specific aspects of nephron function, such as glomerular filtration, blood flow, and proximal and tubular handling of normal and exogenous solutes. A brief summary of clinical tests of renal function is illustrated in Table 6–3.

The clinical tests which appear to have most utility because of past experience and clinical availability are the plasma concentrations of creatinine and urea. Although these values may fall within the normal range in patients with significant renal functional impairment, any patient with advanced renal failure, as measured by other parameters, will have an abnormal plasma value. The concentrating test will frequently show impairment in various nephropathies before significant depression of the GFR with elevation of the serum creatinine is noted. This is apparently due to the remarkable capacity of the remaining viable nephrons to increase in size and compensate for loss of nephron mass.

Other tests of renal tubular function are available, but are reserved for patients with specific problems. Because of special requirements of constant infusions or the measurement of specific chemicals, they are cumbersome for routine use and are most often carried out in research facilities.

Evaluation of the Structure of the Urinary System.   A plain x-ray picture of the abdomen with emphasis on the region of the kidneys, ureters, and bladder (the so-called KUB) is an important first step to subsequent urographic examination. The size and location of the kidneys can often be seen, especially in obese people who have a layer of relatively radiolucent fat surrounding the kidney. Radiopaque stones in the kidneys, ureters, or bladder will be most easily seen before contrast agents are used. Occasionally, a large renal mass or over-distended bladder may be appreciated by this examination.

An *excretory urogram* (commonly miscalled an intravenous pyelogram or IVP) is an extremely useful method for visualizing the kidney and lower urinary tract by radiography. The study is done by an intravenous infusion of a tri-iodinated benzoic acid derivative. The iodine molecule provides radiopacity, while the benzoic acid molecule is rapidly filtered by the kidney. After the intravenous injection of 25 to 30 gm of a contrast agent (Hypaque-50, Renograffin-60 or Conray-60), the drug becomes concentrated in the renal tubules within the first five minutes, providing a nephrogram. Some time later, the contrast agent appears in the collecting system, outlining the renal pelvis, the ureters, and finally the bladder. This ability to visualize the urinary system is dependent on adequate renal function and, to some degree, on the absence of an osmotic or water diuresis which would dilute the contrast agent. Therefore, the best radiograms are obtained in patients with a normal GFR who have been water restricted. It is usually difficult to obtain an adequate study in patients with a BUN greater than 70 mg/100 ml or a plasma creatinine greater than 7 mg/100 ml.

There are many reasons for obtaining an excretory urogram: evaluation for suspected tumor, trauma of the abdomen or pelvis; evaluation of the function and structure of one kidney versus the other; and assessment of the size and capacity of the bladder before and after voiding, and of possible structural damage caused by chronic infection. The technique is also useful in evaluating the position of other abdominal masses by the displacement of the urinary system. Severe allergic reactions to the contrast agents occur about once in 10,000 times. Skin rashes, however, occur more frequently.

The *retrograde pyelogram* is a procedure in which radiopaque agents similar to those used in excretory urography are introduced directly into the urinary tract following cystoscopy and catheterization of the ureters. The technique is useful in providing an intense opacification of the collecting and voiding system where the excretory urogram has been unsuccessful owing to poor renal function.

The *cystogram* obtained as a part of an excretory urogram may not be satisfactory owing to poor opacification or incomplete filling. Controlled bladder filling utilizing a catheter (*retrograde cystogram*) is then necessary for adequate visualization and evaluation of reflux into the ureters from the bladder, which is always an abnormal finding. The male urethra may be examined by the retrograde injection of a contrast agent, although all the information needed is frequently seen in a voiding film after an excretory urogram. When the retrograde urethral injection is combined with cystography, the combined procedure is called *retrograde urethrocystography*. In women and children, the bladder and urethra are often evaluated by *cystourethrography* with or without *cineradiography* to better appreciate the dynamics of micturition.

Special radiographic methods may be used to define the arterial supply (*arteriography*) or the venous system (*venography*) of related or adjacent structures. Their use is confined to special problems of renal blood supply.

Isotope Studies. In addition to conventional urography, procedures for studying renal function and structure by the excretion of chemicals labeled with radioisotopes are also available. Because only trace amounts of chemicals need be given, the danger of hypersensitivity reactions is decreased, and with the use of rapidly decaying isotopes the biological damage from radiation is small. Procedures available include renograms and renal scans. Since the advent of the gamma camera, both of these procedures can be done simultaneously, and a sequential temporal record of events can be recorded. A renogram involves recording radioactivity over each kidney following an intravenous injection of a gamma-ray-emitting labeled substance which is rapidly excreted by the kidney such as ^{125}I-orthoiodohippurate (Hippuran). This technique has been used in part for screening patients for possible renal vascular hypertension. Because Hippuran remains in the kidney such a short period of time, it has not been found useful for obtaining renal scans except when the gamma camera is available. With slower scanning techniques ^{203}Hg-chlormerodrin is used, as it is retained by the renal tubules and enables the renal outlines to be traced by an external counter. Scans may be helpful when the excretory urogram is equivocal in cases of ischemia or space-occupying lesions. It is also useful in determining the presence of functioning tissue mass.

Renal Biopsy. There are four reasons given for performing renal biopsies. First, they are helpful in establishing a histologic diagnosis. Second, a biopsy is frequently useful in estimating prognosis and the potential reversibility or progression of the renal lesion. Third, knowledge of the renal histology may suggest whether treatment will be or has been useful. Fourth, serial histologic evaluations are necessary to establish the natural history of renal diseases. The only absolute contraindication to a biopsy is an uncorrectable bleeding disorder. A solitary kidney and an uncooperative patient may serve as other contraindications. Because the incidence of complications is so low, the biopsy of a solitary kidney is only a relative contraindication if the information that might be gained is considered valuable enough. Biopsies of a single, functioning transplanted kidney have been done frequently to diagnose and study possible graft rejections. Conditions which are associated with an increased morbidity following biopsy are deemed relative contraindications and include renal tumors, large renal cysts, hydronephrosis, perinephric abscesses, severe reduction in blood or plasma volume, severe hypertension, and advanced renal failure with symptoms of uremia.

There are basically two techniques: open and percutaneous biopsy. The percutaneous technique is most common. The open surgical method is necessary only when the percutaneous method has not been successful or when direct visual control of the biopsy site is deemed critical.

The percutaneous technique involves sedation of the patient, infusion of a radiographic contrast agent, visualization of the kidney by use of video-monitored fluoroscopy with the patient in the prone position, local anesthesia of the overlying skin and muscle of the back, and insertion of a biopsy needle under fluoroscopic control. Tissue is commonly obtained for light, electron, and immunofluorescent microscopy.

Cystoscopy is a surgical procedure involving the introduction of a metal tube containing visual apparatus into the bladder through the urethra, which allows the operator to inspect the urethra and bladder. The procedure requires special training and experience in order to minimize trauma and discomfort to the patient. It is performed under local or general anesthesia, depending upon the amount of manipulation required for a particular problem. Following insertion of the cystoscope into the bladder, sterile water is instilled to distend the bladder and to enable direct inspection of the mucosal lining, identification of ureteral orifices, or direct biopsy of suspicious lesions. Utilizing special equipment, calculi may be broken up and extracted from the ureters or bladder, and neoplasms may be resected in a piecemeal fashion. Prostatectomies can also be done by special instruments of this type.

Bladder Catheterization. Although clinicians tend to view the placement of the bladder catheter as only a therapeutic maneuver, it is also a diagnostic test. For example, catheterization may be used to discover the presence of post-voiding residual urine or to obtain bladder urine for culture.

It is often desirable to catheterize the bladder in order to assure good drainage. Good catheter care starts *before* insertion of the catheter. The steps for safe catheterization include the following: (1) insuring patient cooperation by an explanation of the procedure followed by an unhurried reassuring action; (2) obtaining good light and assistance as needed; (3) washing the urethral meatus gently and thoroughly with mild antiseptic and lubricating the urethra generously by injection of 10 to 15 ml of a water-soluble lubricant directly into the urethra, and (4) wearing gloves or passing the catheter with instruments and *being gentle* at all times. The smallest catheter sufficient to do the job is the one that is indicated. A #16 Fr. in the adult male, or a #18 Fr. in the adult female, are average values. Larger sizes may need to be used in the presence of bloody urine with clots.

If frequent catheter irrigation is required, a closed irrigating system is best, and a three way catheter may be desirable. If hand irrigation is necessary, follow aseptic techniques. If an indwelling catheter is placed, the meatus and catheter should be cleansed daily with soap and water to allow free egress of urethral secretions. A high fluid intake is desirable and may help to prevent migration of bacteria contaminants from the urinary receptacle through the drainage tubing into the bladder. To further reduce this chance of bacterial growth, 10 ml of 10% formalin for each liter of container size are introduced into the collection bag daily when the system is emptied. With the aid of such precautions, infections associated with catheter drainage can be kept to a minimum (less than 3%) for short-term drainage and significantly reduced for longer periods.

In order to test the complex reflex arc responsible for normal bladder tone and capacity and to document symptoms of bladder dysfunction, a *cystometrogram* is often used. In this test, a bladder catheter is introduced and used to fill the bladder to a series of given volumes. The intraluminal pressure at which the patient senses a full bladder and begins to contract is noted.

CLINICAL DATA ANALYSIS

The data described in the previous section are important in determining both the presence and type of urinary system problems. Each bit of information must be interpreted in the context of anatomy and physiology. Clinical data analysis is a scientific approach involving observations (subjective and objective) that are used to form a hypothesis, which can be tested by further data collection. Eventually a conclusion is reached, which is called a "working diagnosis."

This section will illustrate, in very simple terms, the logic associated with clinical data analysis. Two clinical problems will be used as models: hematuria and urinary frequency.

Hematuria. The presence of blood in the urine is cause for alarm, as it may be a harbinger of serious disease in the urinary system. Hematuria is called gross or macroscopic when it can be detected by the human eye. In health, red cell excretion is about 3,000/min. Hematuria is macroscopic when more than a million red cells are excreted per minute. Excretion less than this must be detected by occult blood tests or microscopic examination. It is important, at this point, to emphasize that sources of urine contamination with blood should always be considered, and the genital tract (vaginitis or menstruation) in women is always suspect.

Analysis of hematuria is best considered in the setting of the possible causes of this disorder. These are summarized in Table 6–4.

The clinician, in his approach to any medical problem, searches for clues which will help separate the various types of hematuria. For example, most cases of macroscopic hematuria are caused by lesions of the collecting and voiding system, whereas the presence of red cell casts is

A Clinical Approach to Diseases of the Urinary System

Table 6-4. Major Causes of Hematuria.

RENAL
 Infections
 Tumor
 Stones
 Trauma
 Polycystic disease
 Glomerulonephritis
 Infarction
 Sickle cell disease
 Arteritis

COLLECTING AND VOIDING SYSTEM
 Tumor
 Stones
 Infections
 Trauma
 Parasites

ANY SITE IN URINARY SYSTEM
 Disorders of coagulation

strong evidence for glomerulonephritis. A problem solving approach to hematuria, using the presence or absence or red cell casts as an initial decision, is diagrammed in Figure 6–2.

Hematuria from Contamination.

A 65 year old woman being treated for severe headaches was noted to have microscopic hematuria without proteinuria or red cell casts in all voided urine specimens. No other pertinent subjective or objective data were present.

A likely cause of hematuria in any woman is contamination from the genital tract. In order to test this possibility, a catheterized urine sample was obtained without trauma and failed to show hematuria. Thus, the technique of obtaining urine directly from the bladder, especially in women, may help solve a hematuria problem due to contamination from a non-urinary tract source.

Hematuria with Red Cell Casts.

A 45 year old man sought help for an infected and swollen left leg. About one week before, he had lacerated his leg while working. Examination showed cellulitis and edema of the lower leg with lymphadenopathy in the left groin. He was afebrile but had mild leukocytosis. The urine contained protein, red cells, and many red cell casts.

The presence of microscopic hematuria with red cell casts and proteinuria in this man suggests that glomerulonephritis is probably present. The history of an injured leg and the finding of infection suggests that the two problems may be related. It is always possible that the urinary abnormalities preceded the leg infection, and in the absence

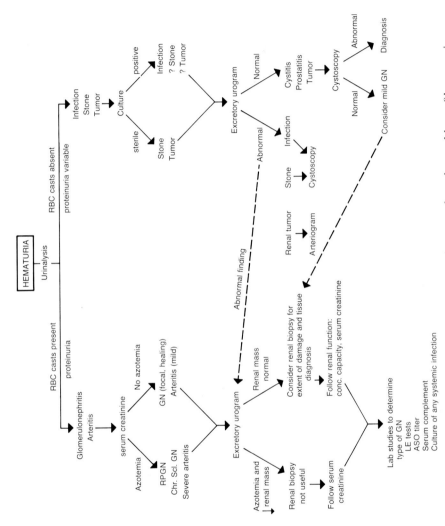

Figure 6–2.   A flow chart depicting a clinical approach to the problem of hematuria.

of a prior urine examination this possibility cannot be excluded. The finding of streptococci in the wound or pharynx and rising titers of antibodies to streptococcal antigens would be helpful in suggesting a relationship to the glomerulonephritis. Other pyogenic infections, such as staphylococci, may also be causally related. The finding of a depressed serum complement titer would be additional evidence of a post-infectious immune complex glomerulonephritis. Finally, a normal excretory urogram would help to eliminate structural abnormalities of the collecting and voiding system as possible additional problems and to give some idea of renal mass. A renal biopsy would further document the renal nature of the disorder, quantitate the degree of injury, and offer some prognostic insight.

Hematuria Without Red Cell Casts.

A 35 year old man was found to have hematuria during an annual physical examination. He was asymptomatic and had no physical abnormalities. He was not taking any drugs regularly. The urine contained red and white cells, but no significant protein. Urine cultures were sterile.

In the absence of symptoms, this patient could have bleeding from any part of the urinary system. A history of colic, passing of gravel, or gout might have suggested lithiasis. Men are rarely asymptomatic with pyogenic urinary tract infection, so this is unlikely; its absence was confirmed by a negative urine culture. However, tuberculosis of the urinary system is possible, and skin testing and urine cultures for tuberculosis should be considered. The problem is best resolved by radiographic studies; if these are negative, then cystoscopy is needed to rule out bladder tumor. If both radiographic and cystoscopic examinations are normal, then the possibility of a focal glomerulonephritis or mild proliferative glomerulitis must be considered. In this particular case, the excretory urogram revealed nephrolithiasis which was investigated and treated surgically.

Frequency, Dysuria.   The urinary bladder is a very distensible structure and may hold 400 to 600 ml. The urge to void, however, is usually noted when approximately one-half this capacity is reached. Normally, the bladder is emptied every 4 to 6 hours, depending on the rate of flow. Thus, any abnormality causing increased irritability of the bladder smooth muscle, such as calculi, inflammation, or neurologic dysfunction, or an increase in urine flow caused by diuretics, compulsive water drinking, or glycosuria, will produce a decrease in effective bladder capacity and more frequent urination. Irritative causes of frequency are usually associated with dysuria. Because diseases of the lower urinary tract are common, frequency and dysuria are typical presenting symptoms for many patients and should alert the physician to careful evaluation of the bladder, urethra, and occasionally the kidney itself.

The major causes of frequency with or without dysuria are listed in Table 6–5.

Table 6–5.   Major Causes of Frequency.

Renal (polyuric syndrome)
  Excessive water ingestion
  Diabetes insipidus
  Nephrogenic diabetes insipidus
  Chronic renal disease
  Diuresis: osmotic (glycosuria, mannitol, etc.) or drugs

Bladder
  Infection
  Stones
  Neurogenic bladder dysfunction
  Chronic interstitial cystitis
  Irradiation injury

Prostate
  Infection: bacterial, non-specific
  Tumor: hyperplasia, cancer

Urethra
  Infection: gonococcal, non-specific
  Stricture
  Meatal stenosis
  Caruncle
  Diverticulum

A logical approach to the problem of frequency and dysuria is to evaluate whether the patient is voiding frequently because of large or small urine volumes. This approach to evaluation is taken in the current schema depicted in Figure 6–3. Several examples of this approach will be presented.

Frequency with Polyuria.

A 45 year old woman noted increasing thirst and frequent urination. There was no discomfort on voiding. Daily urine output exceeded 8 liters. The physical examination and screening laboratory studies were unremarkable.

The symptom of frequency here is clearly related to polyuria. There are no symptoms of urinary tract inflammation or irritation. The main differential diagnosis is whether the polyuria is due to an osmotic diuresis such as glycosuria from uncontrolled diabetes mellitus, a lack of ADH (compulsive water drinking or diabetes insipidus), or renal dysfunction with loss of concentrating capacity such as nephrogenic diabetes insipidus. In this case, the urine osmolality was less than 100 mOsm/L, glycosuria was absent, and a normal fasting and post-prandial blood glucose eliminated diabetes mellitus as a consideration. Further studies revealed an inability to concentrate urine during water deprivation but a response to exogenous ADH, thus suggesting the diagnosis of diabetes insipidus. Careful neurological evaluation revealed a brain tumor in the hypothalamic area.

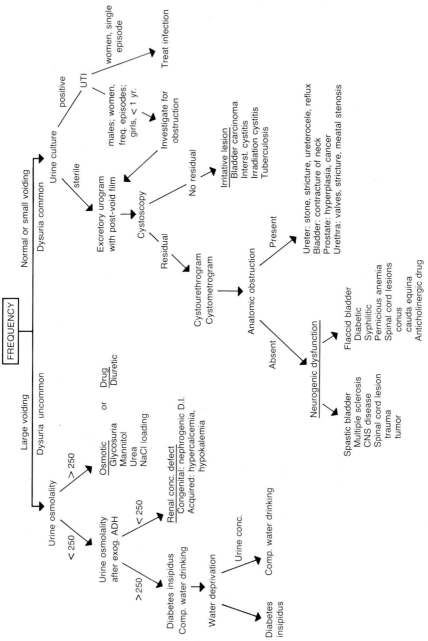

Figure 6–3. A flow chart depicting a clinical evaluation of the problem of urinary frequency.

Frequency with Infection.

A 25 year old woman was seen because of dysuria. She had a history of three similar episodes over the last three years. She was voiding small urine volumes about every hour and was bothered at night as well. Fever and chills were absent, although they had been present with one previous episode. Her current urine contained many leukocytes and bacteria which were visible in an unspun specimen. A mid-stream urine culture contained greater than 10^5 colonies/ml of *E. coli*.

The history of dysuria and frequency with small voidings suggests bladder or urethral irritation or inflammation. The finding of pyuria is confirmatory although (1) it is not always found with urinary tract infections, and (2) in women, pyuria may be seen in voided urine if genital tract leukorrhea exists. If the source of pyuria is in doubt, the bladder should be catheterized in women. The noticeable bacteriuria on urinary microscopy and significant urine culture document the cause of the irritative symptoms.

In view of this patient's history of repeated urinary tract infections, it would be desirable to evaluate the possibility of obstruction. This is particularly true if the infection can be documented to be of the relapsing variety (Chapter 5). If infection is not documented, an entirely different approach to her problem would be required.

Frequency with Obstruction.

A 65 year old man has noted nocturia for several years. There has been no discomfort while urinating, but he has found that it takes longer to start and complete urination than in previous years. He does not feel that he is able to empty his bladder completely and often has the urge to void soon after micturition. On physical examination, a slightly enlarged prostate was found. The serum creatinine and urinalysis are normal and no bacteria were cultured from the urine. An excretory urogram was normal, but the post-voiding film showed significant residual bladder urine.

The symptoms of hesitancy in this man suggest obstruction. The post-voiding film confirms an inability to empty his bladder completely, which is probably due to prostatic hyperplasia. The symptoms of frequency are related to this incomplete bladder emptying, which reduces the effective bladder capacity at which the sensation of fullness and urge to micturate occurs. If residual urine is large and the bladder is overstretched, or if anticholinergic medication is taken which impairs bladder function, the detrusor is unable to empty the bladder and urinary retention ensues. Evaluation of obstruction and his bladder capacity could be accomplished by cystoscopy, cystourethrography, and cystometrograms.

PROGRESSIVE RENAL FAILURE

Gradual renal failure occurs in the course of a large number of diseases, eventually reaching the point where kidney function is inadequate to sustain life. With the loss of functioning nephrons, each remaining nephron must perform more of the homeostatic functions of the kidney. Thus, when 80% of the nephrons have been destroyed, the excretory load of each remaining nephron is increased five-fold. This marked increase in the excretory requirements of remaining nephrons results in abnormalities of function which account in part for many of the aberrations seen in renal failure. In addition, damage to functioning nephrons may result from the underlying disease and further distort renal function. In this section, some of the major abnormalities which are encountered in renal disease will be reviewed, and two current methods of treatment, dialysis and transplantation, will be discussed.

Pathophysiologic Changes Associated with Renal Failure

Renal Concentration and Dilution. Typically, the urine of patients with chronic renal failure has an osmolality near 300 mOsm/Kg (specific gravity about 1.010), which is approximately that of plasma; this reflects a loss of concentrating and dilution capacity. This "fixed" urine osmolality represents (1) a loss of functional concentrating capacity due to structural renal damage, and (2) a response to the large osmotic load, especially of urea, imposed on each remaining nephron. When functional renal mass is reduced to 20% of normal, the amount of urea excreted per nephron is increased five-fold. This situation can be simulated in the normal kidney by infusing urea or other substances which act as osmotic diuretics. As the rate of solute increases, the osmolality of the urine approximates that of plasma. Removal of excess solutes by hemodialysis reveals that the loss of dilutional capacity is only apparent and not real, and is due to the large osmotic diuresis per nephron. However, the concentration capacity remains impaired despite adequate dialysis, and this state is due to structural renal damage from disease. In the normal person, the rate of urine excretion decreases considerably at night. In renal failure, however, the constant osmotic diuresis results in a relatively constant rate of urine formation throughout the day and night, resulting in nocturia, a common symptom in this condition.

Sodium Excretion. Normally, about 99% of the filtered sodium is reabsorbed in the nephron. If this situation continued in advanced renal failure with a normal salt intake, the patient would rapidly develop severe saline excess. Fortunately, the diseased kidney adapts to the situation by decreasing the percentage of sodium reabsorbed per nephron to 80% or less of the filtered load. By so doing, it is able to excrete the amount of salt ingested each day and maintain homeostasis. At some point in decreasing renal function, sodium excretion cannot adapt to intake, and unless ingestion is restricted edema and hypertension will occur.

Potassium Excretion. Despite the fact that the potassium excretory load per nephron is markedly increased in renal failure, potassium excess is seldom seen. In this situation, potassium clearance exceeds that of GFR as long as oliguria is not present. When urine flow is severely restricted, potassium excretion is impaired and potassium excess may occur.

Water Balance. As described elsewhere, sensitive control of water balance is achieved by means of the cybernetic mechanisms related to thirst and ADH. In chronic renal failure, thirst continues to exert control over water balance and is adequate to compensate in most patients for loss of the renal regulatory mechanism of dilution and concentration. For this reason, disorders of water balance are uncommon even in the presence of severe renal damage.

Acid-Base Balance. The pathophysiology of chronic metabolic acidosis which occurs in renal failure is discussed in Chapter 4.

Phosphate and Calcium Balance. Bone disease, a common complication of chronic renal failure, usually takes the form of both secondary hyperparathyroidism and osteomalacia. Unfortunately, bone disease may progress despite otherwise adequate dialysis, but it is less of a problem when a good renal graft is obtained. The problem appears to be due, in part, to an insensitivity to the usual amounts of dietary vitamin D, resulting in greatly decreased absorption of calcium from the gut and in changes in bone cell metabolism resulting in osteomalacia. Vitamin D resistance can be demonstrated early in renal failure and is related to a change in its metabolism and cellular action. In addition, an increase in plasma parathyroid hormone level develops early in renal failure and is responsible for some of the severe bone changes (osteitis fibrosa cystica).

Anemia. Chronic renal disease usually results in the development of anemia. The pathogenesis of the anemia is related to the failure of renal excretion of toxic metabolic products and a decrease in renal production of erythropoietic factor.

The uremic syndrome produced by renal failure is associated with increased blood loss (usually via the GI tract), a decreased red cell life span, and ineffective red cell production. These changes are only moderately stressful and could easily be met by a normal bone marrow. However, the major defect in the uremic patient is an inability of the bone marrow to respond with compensatory hyperplasia. This failure of compensation is due both to a decreased production of erythropoietic factor by the diseased kidney and to an impaired response by the bone marrow.

Protein Metabolism. Many of the symptoms of uremia, such as malaise, anorexia, nausea, and vomiting, which are non-specific but very distressing to patients, are related to retention of products of protein metabolism. Urea is the most easily measured of these substances, and the BUN thus serves as a guide to the rate of protein metabolism relative to renal function. High urea levels alone may account for some uremic symptoms, but other metabolites also contribute substantially to the symptomatology. By reducing protein intake and thus reducing the body levels of these metabolites, the gastroinestinal symptoms of uremia can be ameliorated. Most patients can adjust well to a low protein diet containing 30 to 40 gm daily of high quality protein.

Patient Treatment in End-Stage Renal Disease

Hemodialysis. The artificial kidney, or hemodialyzer, was first conceived by Abel, Rountree, and Turner in 1912. It took three decades and three events before the artificial kidney was first applied to man. Cellophane had to be developed by industry to provide a cheap, readily available membrane. A suitable anticoagulant, heparin, had to be discovered, and the right combination of machinery had to be devised by Kolff before the first clinical artificial kidney was used in 1944. From then until 1960, the artificial kidney was used to treat only patients with reversible renal failure, since surgical implantation of cannulas (tubes) in blood vessels was required for each treatment. In 1960, Quinton, Dillard, and Scribner developed the arteriovenous shunt, which permitted more or less permanent implantation of cannulas and made repetitive hemodialysis possible.

An artificial kidney is a device in which blood and dialysis fluid flow at high rates in opposite directions, separated by a thin, semipermeable membrane. The two basic processes which take place inside the hemodialyzer are diffusion and ultrafiltration of solutes and fluid through the pores of the membrane. Diffusion can occur in either direction. Diffusion from blood to dialysate is exhibited by urea, creatinine, phosphate, sulfate, and potassium. Diffusion from blood to dialysate takes place because of the high concentration of these molecules bombarding the membrane on the blood side and their absence on the dialysate side. Diffusion from dialysate to blood is exhibited in the correction of metabolic acidosis, which is accomplished by the use of hydrogen acceptors such as bicarbonate or acetate ions in the dialysis fluid in concentrations high enough to diffuse into the blood passing through the dialyzer. On the other hand, the control of water and sodium transfer during hemodialysis is accomplished by ultrafiltration. A low dialysate sodium concentration cannot be used to produce a diffusion gradient to remove sodium because water, which moves faster than sodium, would leave the dialysis fluid more rapidly than sodium would enter the dialysate, producing a positive water transfer to the patient with the production of severe water excess.

Hospital or medical center use of the artificial kidney, formerly predominant, recently has been abandoned because of its enormous cost and has been replaced by home use. Three times weekly over-night dialysis will restore most patients to good health. Obviously, the effort, expense, and emotional strain involved in operation of a potentially lethal device at home represents a less than ideal solution to the problem.

Renal Homotransplantation. The ideal treatment for end-stage renal disease would be a new kidney, natural or artificial. The only reliable implantable source of renal function currently is a renal graft. The level of renal function achieved by a graft is generally superior to that provided by hemodialysis. It should be realized, however, that transplantation is restricted to a smaller group of patients than is dialysis. In particular, patients whose renal disorder is caused by systemic disease (diabetes mellitus, atherosclerosis) are not acceptable candidates at the present time for transplantation. Because of the effect of immunosuppressive drugs on the body defense mechanisms, it is mandatory that no patient receiving transplantation have a urinary system infectious process. This excludes patients with lower urinary tract disease and associated infection. If the infection can be eliminated, these patients can be successfully treated with renal transplantation.

In human transplant terminology, tissue and organ grafts are classified as either autografts or homografts (also called isografts or allografts). Autografts are grafts between one portion of an individual's body and another portion of that same individual's body. These grafts, if performed properly, will survive indefinitely without any special treatment. Homografts, isografts, or allografts, on the other hand, are grafts which are taken from members of the same species who are *not* genetically identical. Unless special efforts are made to suppress the immunological response of the homograft recipient by irradiation or drugs, the graft will be rejected within 7 to 10 days.

It has been clearly demonstrated in human transplantation that kidneys which are provided by family members are grafted more successfully than kidneys which are taken from unrelated individuals. With current methods of treatment, a kidney taken from a family member has approximately a 90% chance of functioning after one year and an 88% chance of functioning after two years. Furthermore, experience which extends to over seven years shows that, despite the shortcomings of the initial immunosuppressive regimens and lack of histocompatibility typing, patients who have kidneys from blood relatives have a 60% chance of surviving seven years. In contrast, only 55% of those kidneys donated by unrelated individuals will be functioning after one year and 48% after two years. Thus, there is a clear-cut difference in outlook depending upon the donor-recipient relationship. Unfortunately, the related donor source of renal grafts is limited. The unrelated or cadaveric graft offers a potential unlimited resource if the problems of histocompatibility and immunological tolerance can be solved.

BIBLIOGRAPHY

Chapter 1

Hayes, R. M.: Dynamics of body water and electrolytes, in *Clinical Disorders of Fluid and Electrolyte Metabolism*, ed. by Maxwell, M. H., and Kleeman, C. R., McGraw-Hill, Inc., N.Y., 1972. Pp. 1–44.

Moore, F. D., Olesen, H., McMurrey, J. D., Parker, H. V., Ball, M. R., and Boyden, C. M.: *The Body Cell Mass*, W. B. Saunders Co., Philadelphia, 1963.

Pitts, R. F.: *Physiology of the Kidney and Body Fluids*, Yearbook Medical Publishers Inc., Chicago, 1968. Pp. 22–43.

Chapter 2

Bulger, R. E.: The urinary system, in *Histology*, 3rd Ed., ed. by Greep, R. O., and Weiss, L., McGraw-Hill, N.Y., 1973.

Müllendorff, W. Von: Der Ex-Kretionsapparat, "Handbüch der mikroskopischen Anatomie des Menschen," Vol. 7, pt. 1, Springer-Verlag OHG, Berlin, 1930.

Hepinstall, R. H.: *Pathology of the Kidney*, Little Brown & Co., Boston, 1966. Pp. 1–62.

Pitts, R. F.: *Physiology of the Kidney and Body Fluids*, Chicago, Yearbook Medical Publishers Inc., 1968. Pp. 13–21, 44–219, 252–256.

Wesson, L. G.: *Physiology of the Human Kidney*, Grune & Stratton, N.Y., 1969.

Windhager, E. E.: *Micropuncture Techniques and Nephron Function*, Appleton-Century-Crofts, N.Y., 1968.

Simpson, D. P.: Control of Hydrogen Ion Homeostasis and Renal Acidosis. Medicine *50*:503–541, 1971.

Vander, A. J.: Control of Renin Release. Physiology Review *47*:359–382, 1967.

Kiil, F.: Physiology of the renal pelvis and ureter, in *Urology*, ed. by Campbell, M. F., and Harrison, J. H., W. B. Saunders Co., Philadelphia, 1970. Pp. 68–104.

Boyarsky, S. and Ruskin, H.: Physiology of the bladder, in *Urology*, ed. by Campbell, M. F., and Harrison, J. H., W. B. Saunders Co., Philadelphia, 1970. Pp. 105–136.

Chapter 3

Fisher, J. W., and Cafruny, E. J.: *Renal Pharmacology*, Appleton-Century-Crofts, N.Y., 1971.

Kleeman, C. R.: Water metabolism, in *Clinical Disorders of Fluid and Electrolyte Metabolism*, ed. by Maxwell, M. H., and Kleeman, C. R., McGraw-Hill, N.Y., 1972. Pp. 215–296.

Reidenberg, M. M.: *Renal Function and Drug Action*, W. B. Saunders Co., Philadelphia, 1971.

Mudge, G. H.: Diuretics and other agents employed in the mobilization of edema fluid, in *The Pharmacological Basis of Therapeutics*, 4th Ed., ed. by Goodman, L. S., and Gilman, A., Macmillan Co., N.Y., 1970.

Chapter 4

Scribner, B. H., ed., *University of Washington Teaching Syllabus for the Course on Fluid and Electrolyte Balance*, University of Washington Press, 1969.

Maxwell, M. H., and Kleeman, C. R., eds., *Clinical Disorders of Fluid and Electrolyte Metabolism*, McGraw-Hill, N.Y., 1972.

Chapter 5

Campbell, M. F., and Bunge, R. G., Embryology and anomalies of the urogenital tract, in *Urology*, ed. by Campbell, M. F., and Harrison, J. H., W. B. Saunders Co., Philadelphia, 1970. Pp. 1379–1671.

Hepinstall, R. H.: *Pathology of the Kidney*, Little Brown & Co., Boston, 1966. Pp. 63–117.

Emmett, J. L., and Witten, D. F.: Congenital anomalies, in *Clinical Urography*, W. B. Saunders Co., 1971. Vol. III, Pp. 1349–1597.

Strauss, M. B., and Welt, L. G.: *Diseases of the Kidney*, Little Brown & Co., Boston, 1971. Pp. 373–636, 1223–1274.

Dodge, W. F., et al.: Post-streptococcal glomerulonephritis (a prospective study in childhood). New Eng. J. Med., *286*:273–278, 1972.

254

Baldwin, D. S., et al.: The clinical course of the proliferative and membranous forms of lupus nephritis. Ann. Intern. Med. 73:929, 1970.

Morel-Maroger, L., et al.: Glomerular abnormalities in non-systemic diseases. Amer. J. Med. 53:170, 1972.

Laragh, J. H.: Ed. Symposium on Hypertension, Mechanisms and Management. Amer. J. Med. 52:565–678, 1972.

Muehrcke, R. C.: *Acute Renal Failure: Diagnosis and Treatment*, C. V. Mosby, St. Louis, 1969.

Hinman, F.: Pathophysiology of urinary obstruction, in *Urology*, ed. by Campbell, M. F., and Harrison, J. H., W. B. Saunders Co., Philadelphia, 1970. Pp. 313–348.

Smith, D. R.: Chapters 12 and 17 in *General Urology*, Lange Medical Publications, Los Altos, California, 1969.

Freedman, L. R.: Urinary tract infection, pyelonephritis and other forms of chronic interstitial nephritis, in *Diseases of the Kidney*, ed. by Strauss, M. B. and Welt, L. G., Little Brown & Co., Boston, 1971.

Smith, L. H., Jr.: Symposium on Stones. Amer. J. Med. 45:649–788, 1968.

Campbell, M. F., and Harrison, J. H., eds.: *Urology*, W. B. Saunders Co., Philadelphia, 1970.

Chapter 6

Epstein, F. H.: Approach to the patient with renal disease, in *Harrison's Principles of Internal Medicine*, 6th Ed., McGraw-Hill, N.Y., 1971, Pp. 1383–1384.

Leader, A. J., and Carlton, C. E., Jr.: Urologic diagnosis and the urologic examination, in *Urology*, ed. by Campbell, M. F., and Harrison, J. H., W. B. Saunders Co., Philadelphia, 1970.

Lippman, R. W.: *Urine and Urine Sediment. A Practical Manual and Atlas*, Charles C Thomas, Springfield, Illinois, 1951.

Kark, R. M., Lawrence, J. R., Pollak, V. E., Pirani, C. L., Muehrcke, R. C., and Silva, H.: *A Primer of Urinalysis*, 2nd Ed., Harper and Row, N.Y., 1963.

Atkins, R. C., Leonard, C. D., and Scribner, B. H.: Management of chronic renal failure. Disease-A-Month, March 1971.

INDEX

256